BRAIN EXERCISES FOR SENIORS

PUZZLES TO KEEP YOUR MIND YOUNG AND NIMBLE

D1403693

By

Jenny Patterson and The Puzzler

TABLE OF CONTENTS

INTRODUCTION

This book contains a variety of puzzles designed to exercise the brain and mind. In fact, we consider it part of a brain fitness routine.

Experts around world have known for some time that working the brain with challenging puzzles helps keep the thought processes younger and nimbler.

We all know about the benefits of physical exercise; bigger muscles, increased agility, and endurance. The benefits of brain exercises may not, at first, be quite as obvious, but the changes these create in cognitive ability can change lives.

Individuals of all ages need to keep learning new things, exploring challenges, and solving puzzles to stay young, alert, and at their mental best.

The large print and easy-to-read formatting in this book make it perfect for seniors and for anyone wanting to avoid the eye-strain of the small type found in most such books.

Happy Solving!

Jenny Patterson & The Puzzler

Dear Fellow Puzzle Lovers,

Thank you for purchasing this book. I hope it brings you hours of enjoyment.

As a small publishing company, reviews are the lifeblood of our continued success. If you could take a few minutes to leave us a review on Amazon it would be greatly appreciated.

www.oldtownpublishing.com/reviews

Thank you, Jenny

CROSSWORDS

CROSSWORD PUZZLE #1

PUZZLE #1 CLUES

Across

1 _____Kingdom - Disneyland

3 Feeble

6 Leave out

8 Tokyo's country

10 Sum up

11 Beats scissors

13 Slowly, but surely

16 Outs opposite

17 Hurricane center

19 Goes with chips

20 Subjects

21 Bound

22 Comic strip

23 Sinatra's 'way'

24 So very much

25 Nope, not, negatory

26 Wonder

28 Mad scientist's milieu

29 Nest resident

31 Historic period

33 Aye; affirmative

34 A Cub Scout group

35 Belonging to

36 Wife of dad

Down

1 Army rank

2 Customary; common

3 Tied the knot

4 Parcel of land

5 Hardwood shade provider

7 Old time Uber

9 A must for border crossing

12 Take it easy

14 Reliable

15 What today will be tomorrow

18 All the people

19 Adorned

23 Lots, oodles

27 Level, equal

30 Do this on a green light

32 "I think therefore I____"

CROSSWORD PUZZLE #2

6. OMIT

CROSSWORD PUZZLE #2
CLUES

Across

1 Canvas holder

3 Friends to pots

5 Hello

6 Sherlock's delight

7 Dismal

9 Grouping

10 Deep blue

11 Tack on

12 Santa's helper

13 Departed

14 Stretchy

16 Fashioned

20 Freezing cold

21 Pointed

22 Listening devices

23 Tinted

25 Rocklike

26 Table support

27 Negative

28 Distribute cards

29 A breakfast staple

Down

1 Book of knowledge

2 Goes back and forth

3 Outstanding

4 Declare

5 Paused

6 Informal

7 Mom's mom

8 Making, often in a factory

15 Catch sight of

17 It stands for something

18 Euphoric

19 Make longer

20 Exists

22 Outer limit

24 Total

25 Therefore

CROSSWORD PUZZLE #3

CROSSWORD PUZZLE #3
CLUES

Across

1 Kind of life form

5 Coffee or tea container

7 Years of life

8 Largest continent

9 Not allowed

11 One House of Congress

15 In addition to

16 You and me

17 An oinkster

18 Therefore

20 Verbal communication

22 In the event that

23 The 'x' in 2X4

24 To exist

25 Artist's loft

27 Mob tattletale

29 Partners with fro

30 Young fellow

32 Pens; writes

33 Comes from

34 Gratitude

Down

1 Used to step up or down

2 Heads a committee

3 Too much

4 Spider's creation

6 Act as if

7 I think therefore I _____

10 Framed in a museum

12 People next door

13 Adjust to new conditions

14 Creative thought

16 Rain blocker

19 Belief

21 Places

26 Bear's home

28 Yellow picker-upper

31 A small plunge

32 Cold water for skating

CROSSWORD PUZZLE #4

CROSSWORD PUZZLE #4
CLUES

Across

1 Golf average

2 Stuff bread is made of

4 Sentence pause

7 Holds a dinner place

10 Uncooked

12 Incredible

14 Recurring at a normal rate

17 Clumsy boat

19 Indicates choice

20 Sand hill often enjoyed by buggies

21 Shed tears

22 Expressing the negative

24 ____ upon a time

25 Requests your presence

27 Act

29 Boy child

31 Polish

33 Acquire

34 Lubricated

35 Adore

Down

1 Two lines that don't meet

3 Foul-smelling

4 Overcame

5 Belongst to me

6 Taking away

8 Action word

9 Menaced

11 You and I

13 Very first stages

15 Quote by rote

16 Up and down toys

18 Next to

23 Mary's follower

26 Presidential block

28 On the other hand

29 The girl

30 Bird that gives a hoot

32 Work with

CROSSWORD PUZZLE #5

CROSSWORD PUZZLE #5
CLUES

Across

1 Region of U.S. includes Florida

5 Play on words

7 Night flyer

9 ___ bat; waiting to hit

10 Looked at

12 Atop

14 Exact, said of memory

16 Mouth part, covers teeth

18 Insulting

21 Became aware of through sound

22 Destroy a pencil mark

23 Pizza portions

25 Causing the most laughter

27 Mouthy

28 Move quickly on foot

29 Stand out

31 Perhaps yes, perhaps no

Down

1 Hair soap

2 Direction of the sky from earth

3 Brand message

4 No winner and no loser

5 Something added before (a word)

6 Nay

8 What person

11 Alps skier's runway

13 Snooze

15 Period when dinosaurs roamed

17 In the event that

19 Rate of recurrence

20 Wrist jewelry

24 That girl

26 On a gift tag

30 That thing

CROSSWORD PUZZLE #6

CROSSWORD PUZZLE #6
CLUES

Across

1 Originate

4 Movements of the ocean

8 From this day forward

9 Received from parents

11 Apple, cherry, or pumpkin

12 Panes of glass on cars

14 Exciting experienced

15 A ship's staff

16 Exact, said of precision

17 In this way

19 Light switch setting

20 Swinging fence part

22 Ardent admirer

23 Symbol for niobium

24 Targets for Botox

27 Every one

28 Forks over the sheckles

Down

1 Environmental management

2 Better to see you with

3 Three-cornered

4 Sticky roof mender

5 Sentence ender

6 Melancholy

7 Talking softly

8 A one-footed jump

10 Infinite

12 In a marvelous way

13 Outstanding

14 Weapons

18 Belongs to us

21 Abbr. for addiction support group

22 Crafty critter

25 Take a snooze

26 Utter

27 Washington's chopping tool

CROSSWORD PUZZLE #7

CROSSWORD PUZZLE #7
CLUES

Across

1 Absorb text

3 Weapon of Indiana Jones

6 Try for a job

9 Flock tender

11 Morning moisture

13 Smallest bit of matter

14 Cinderella's prince

16 Put on

18 Formally present

21 Flip or throw

22 Lively and sprightly

23 Appropriate

24 Goes with vinegar on salad

25 Whoosh across the snow or water

26 Ocean floater

28 Metal rope

29 Consumes food

30 Green soup

31 By its very nature

Down

2 Objective

3 Existed

4 Pirate's pet

5 Ill at ease

7 A cliff shelf

8 Served at tea time

10 Deeply distressing

12 Military conflict

15 Synthetic

16 Sharp humor

17 Without qualification

19 Cosmos

20 Breakfast order

24 Works of Puccini

25 Dance move

27 Feels painful

CROSSWORD PUZZLE #8

CROSSWORD PUZZLE #8
CLUES

Across

1 Smarts

7 Toothy carpentry tool

8 Marvelously

11 Member of Congress

13 Like that

15 The eye has it

17 In that way

18 Beside, next to

19 Green citrus fruit

20 A red fruit used in jam

21 Usually

23 Bar or block

24 Panache

27 Tightly packed

29 deep mouth-open sighing

Down

2 Daily journals of current events

3 Hit the runway

4 Organ for hearing

5 Carefully

6 Blue expanse above

8 Wheeled garden carrier

9 Chow down

10 Untruths

11 Plato's ideal government

12 Power to control

14 Presentation to a deity

16 Rodeo dudes

22 Elderly

25 Attempt

26 Not high or tall

28 Denial

CROSSWORD PUZZLE #9

CROSSWORD PUZZLE #9
CLUES

Across

1 British bar

3 Soft head resters

8 Famously neutral country

12 Magazine displayer

13 Line goes round and round

14 Masticated

16 Did laps in water

17 Car filler

18 Nice places for wine

19 Radio noise

20 Sound teeth make in the cold

22 Petrol

23 Regrettably

25 Hit's opposite

26 Butter serving

Down

1 Like a crossword

2 American pub

3 Vegetable in a pod

4 Showed the way

5 Belonging to

6 Nick - for one

7 Varied mix

8 Vehicle in space

9 Mendacity

10 Mother of Invention

11 Now and then

12 Place to eat

15 How to get there

21 Sensitive

24 A little bite

CROSSWORD PUZZLE #10

CROSSWORD PUZZLE #10
CLUES

Across

1 Theatrical

5 Once around the track

7 Too bad

9 Sleepy rooms

10 Nightingale or Barton for e.g.

11 Unexpectedly

12 Existed

13 Tick tock of the clock

15 Large period of history

16 Grown up puppy

18 Unwell

20 Woodcutters tool

22 Polliwog

25 Humble home or hovel

26 Look to the sunrise here

28 New Jersey Basketball

29 Bone photos

30 Luggage ID

31 Not this

Down

1 Dress in

2 Expressed regrets

3 Like a painter

4 Television choices

6 Checks for balances?

7 Comprehension

8 Audio instrument

9 Below floor level

12 The two of us

14 My way or the____

17 Pay dirt

19 Most recent

21 Got acquainted

23 Solemn promise

24 Highest die roll

27 Yacht spot

CROSSWORD PUZZLE #11

CROSSWORD PUZZLE #11
CLUES

Across

2 Warning of danger or harm
7 Remains after fire
8 Directed above
9 Applaud
10 Sodium to a chemist
11 With a favorable outcome
13 A thing
14 Aluminum to a chemist
15 as a companion
16 Between 're' and 'fa'
17 Responsibility
19 Egg on
21 By and by
22 Secret agent
23 Whichever
24 Finis, no more
27 Rested on your rump
28 Perform
30 Play performers
32 A little lie teller
34 Limerick people
35 Change used to display a buffalo

36 Silicon symbol
37 Navigating the deep blue waters
38 She sheep

Down

1 Center for trade
2 Day for Thanksgiving
3 Particularly
4 Taken from place to place
5 Anger
6 Partner of ladies
12 Shape
13 Types of commercial production
18 Playthings
20 Receive a throw
25 Eat like a rabbit
26 Auto
29 Derived or coming from
31 Belted one out
33 Otherwise

CROSSWORD PUZZLE #12

CROSSWORD PUZZLE #12
CLUES

Across

1 Eye drop

5 Humans

7 Symbol for iridium

8 Dominate and overcome

10 Unruly group

11 Put in position

12 Enemies of "The Sharks"

13 Comes after La in the scale

14 Unclear

15 Kind of a deal

16 Become aware of

19 Crossing at right angles

21 Move along

23 Abbr. for Alaska

24 A honey buzzer

27 Dropped swiftly

28 A transport to Venus

29 Beaver's work product

Down

1 Down a football player

2 Irksome

3 Rural area

4 Pen point

5 Biased

6 Removes contents

9 Causing unease

15 Loud noise

17 At the center of an atom

18 Made bigger

20 Needed to play oboe or clarinet

22 Must pay

24 A Greyhound

25 Historic period

26 Fire leftovers

27 Explode a balloon

CROSSWORD PUZZLE #13

CROSSWORD PUZZLE #13
CLUES

Across

1 Little cat feet

6 Tin and Lead for e.g.

8 Yours and mine

9 Cover for a jar

10 Animal famous at Christmas

12 Peculiar

13 Before recorded time

14 Inquires

16 Shenanigan

17 Fruit with a tricky peel

19 Home of the hula

20 Chef

22 Inactive

24 Declare

25 Happy

27 Circles, squares, or triangles, e.g.

Down

1 An extremely accurate memory

2 Planet

3 Look for

4 Almost an island

5 Traits

6 Withstand

7 Witness

11 Entance to a room

15 Walloped

17 Heavily satirical

18 "Negatory"

21 Olive or canola for e.g.

23 Belt guide

24 Came to rest on the rear

25 Monopoly corner

26 Before noon

CROSSWORD PUZZLE #14

CROSSWORD PUZZLE #14
CLUES

Across

2 Thicker half of half and half

4 Situated

5 In a direction above

6 Owned by me

7 Exposed film

8 Do_____others (Biblical phrase)

9 Foreign or strange

11 Partner with chips

12 Purposefully

14 Exists

15 Sweet fruit eaten with cream

17 Outer limits

20 Home to Big Ben

22 Verbal response to pain

23 Elementary

24 Thee or thou

25 Singing the story

26 Head covering

27 Partner with neither

28 Every bit

Down

1 Beach hut

2 Chats

3 Growing in amount

4 Tongues

6 Sea surrounding Sicily

8 Without clothing

10 Part of FBI

13 Statute

16 Tin star

18 Equivalent

19 The two

21 What the nose knows

24 Affirmative vote

CROSSWORD PUZZLE #15

CROSSWORD PUZZLE #15
CLUES

Across

2 More or less

8 A person

9 Reject

12 Moved quickly on foot

13 Onward's partner

15 Tagged player

16 Even

17 Seat for two

18 911 responder

19 Frozen spike

20 Car stopper

21 Capri, for one

22 Universal Time

24 Perimeter

25 Greater than drizzling

27 A musical tine

29 Condemn

32 Barbecue site

Down

1 Possesses

2 Management

3 Effective

4 Crushing

5 Central

6 Symbol for titanium

7 Little dog sound

10 Foil

11 Without restraint

12 Brought back to mind

14 Bringing forth a baby

23 Tore

26 Not one

28 Attempt

30 Plow puller

31 Providing

CROSSWORD PUZZLE #16

CROSSWORD PUZZLE #16
CLUES

Across

1 A collection of facts
7 Expression of surprise
8 "Scram"
9 Bounding gait
10 In a direction toward
12 Biblical pronoun
13 Setting for "The Jungle Book"
14 Tiny worker
16 Consume
17 Swapped names
19 Hamlet's home
20 Deli purchase
21 Terminates
23 Thesaurus entry
25 Bind
26 1980's TV alien
27 Where a pupil resides
29 Legislative bodies in Europe
32 Plus
34 Old day partnering with feathers

Down

2 Butterfly catcher
3 Thousand thousand
4 Jailed
5 Silent assent
6 Lowest card
8 Germanium symbol
10 Agatha Christie's little indians
11 On and on and on
12 Voting days
14 Like the Dead Sea Scrolls
15 Frog of the future
17 The boot in the sea
18 Rug rats
22 Most secure
24 Belongs to me
28 Measure of corn
30 Arsenic to a chemist
31 Artificial intelligence
33 Perform

CROSSWORD PUZZLE #17

CROSSWORD PUZZLE #17
CLUES

Across

1 The pause that refreshes a sentence
4 Fruit drinks
7 Stop color
10 A sailor
12 Take to court
13 Policy subject
14 Gave meaning to
15 How you get the tail on the donkey
16 That girl
17 Enough
19 Combustible car power
21 Flute or lute, e.g.
22 Neptune's realm
24 Have dinner
26 Book of words
31 After la

Down

1 Was able
2 Unmoving
3 Reaches
5 Legal matter
6 Using vocal cords
8 A let down
9 Intersecting at right angles
11 Declaration of July 1776
15 Aviators
18 fish guides
20 Years of existence
22 Unhappy
23 Curved line
25 Ball and strike caller
27 That is, abbr.
28 Bathroom staple
29 Kipling classic
30 Like Christopher or Nick

CROSSWORD PUZZLE #18

CROSSWORD PUZZLE #18
CLUES

Across

1 Doctor

4 Existed

7 Land named for Vespucci

8 Parental sister

9 Black, sticky substance

10 Convict quickly and unfairly

12 Pilotless plane

14 Of the moon

15 Science of farming

16 Harley Davidson bike

17 Scientific tests

20 Caesar's nationality

22 Pagination of a document

24 Comfort or support

25 "Dead _____" - without expression

26 No winner and no loser

27 Almost 40 inches

28 Initials of a famous railway

30 Chop, chop

31 Sneaky

Down

1 Type of clock

2 An important point in arithmatic

3 Up to the job

4 Kind of a blanket

5 Leave you in stitches

6 Attaboy

10 Save from peril

11 Must haves

13 Patent candidates

18 Frog's hangout

19 Timid, mild

21 Identifies

23 Precious stone

25 A shade of green

27 Owned by me

29 3.14159

CROSSWORD PUZZLE #19

CROSSWORD PUZZLE #19
CLUES

Across
1 Didn't feel well
2 Mail deliverers
6 Sometimes bubble
7 Classy diners
9 A turn
10 Precedes Lanka
11 Excuses or reasons
13 Once existed
14 Dazzling display
15 Top of a jar
16 Give up the ghost
17 Where X might mark the spot
19 First Lady of earth
20 Foot warmers
22 Function
24 Colored
25 Those people
27 Morsel
28 Unit of energy

30 On the fringes
31 Calendar units
32 Interjection of annoyance

Down
1 Pitcher's pride
2 Intertwine
3 Encircle
4 Lion's pride
5 Double path for air
6 Cake used to build a house
7 Brought to light
8 Word units
9 Substitute
12 Pointed out
13 Baby carriers
18 Cherry, berry, or pumpkin
21 A girl child
23 Stand up entrance
26 Affirmative
29 Get into motion

CROSSWORD PUZZLE #20

CROSSWORD PUZZLE #20
CLUES

Across

1 Language of Rembrandt

4 House warmer

7 Pictures used to explain

10 Bowling target

11 Injured parties

12 Like a lemon

13 The loneliest number

14 In a manner undisturbed

16 Centers of higher learning

18 Campus groups

20 Of greatest size

22 A satellite of Jupiter

23 Alleviate

25 Delaware abbr.

26 As well

27 A type of hockey

28 Put down

29 Bride's new title

30 Slang for really liked

Down

2 First note of a major scale

3 Chopper

4 Celebrations

5 Senora Peron

6 1901 to 2000 for e.g.

7 What PIs do

8 In good repute

9 Rude remarks

10 Say the word

15 Any one of these in a storm

17 Outer portion

19 To get with great effort

21 Done

24 Help

26 Symbol for Thorium

27 Exists

SUDOKU PUZZLES

PUZZLE 1

5	1	6	8		2			
9	2	7			3	6	1	8
			7		1			2
	7	1	2		9	3		
8		9		7		4	2	
4	5			1	8	9		7
	4	3			6	8		9
2	6	8	9			1		4
7	9		1	8	4	2		

3	9	7	4			5		
1		5		2	7	4		3
4				8			7	1
		2	7				4	6
7	6	9	8	5		3		2
8	3			6	1		9	
2		3					8	4
	4		6		2			
	7	1	5	4	8	2		9

PUZZLE 3

8			5	9		3	2	6
5	6		3			4	8	7
	3		6		8			
		1		3	7			4
6	2	8			1	7		9
	7	4	8	6			5	
	9			2		5	4	
1	8		9		5			3
		5	7	8	3	6		

PUZZLE 4

			1			3	9	
1	3	5	9		7			4
9	8			4	6	1		
	7		6	9	1		5	2
6	5	9	8	2	3			7
8	2	1	5			9		
	6	4		3	9	7	8	1
			7	1			4	
2	1		4	6		5		

PUZZLE 5

4		3	8			9	6	
	9		6		4	1	3	8
8			9					4
	3		2			6	7	
6			7	5		2	4	
5		2		4		8	9	
9	4	6	5		1	3	8	2
2			3	8	9		1	6
		8	4	6	2	7		

PUZZLE 6

	1		4	7			9	6
6		7	2	3	9			
4	9	8	1			7		3
8	4		7		2			
	2	9		4	3	6	1	
5	3	6						4
		5		2		1	3	
3	6				7		8	5
			3			9	6	

PUZZLE 7

			6					8
8	2	6		3		7		
4	9			5	7	3	2	
1	8				3	9		2
	7			2		1	6	
6	5		1		4			
3	6	8	2	4	1		7	9
	4		3	7				
2		7					4	

PUZZLE 8

			4			1	5	
		3	9	5	7	4	6	8
		5	2				3	9
	7		5				4	
9				1	8		2	7
5	2		7	9			1	3
			8	4	9		7	
3		7	1			6		4
1	4	9	3	7				5

PUZZLE 9

8		5	4	9			6	1
2	1	9	6		8	7	5	4
6						2	8	9
			3				9	2
7	9	4		2				
5				8		6	4	
			9		1	4		5
	2	1	8	5		9	7	
				7	4	8	1	

PUZZLE 10

6	9	5	7				2	3
8			4	3				
4				5	9		8	7
						9		
	3	8		2	1			6
	7		6	4			1	
	5	1	3	6			7	
		9	5	8			6	
7				9	2	3	5	4

PUZZLE 11

7				4	9	6	5	1
4	1				5	8		
				8	2	9		4
		1	2	6	7	3		5
			9	5				2
5	6		4	3	8			7
	3	4		9			1	8
		6			4		3	9
			8	2	3	7	4	6

PUZZLE 12

1			6	2	5	8	9	3
8	9	3		4	7			6
	2	5		9		7		
	8	4	5	7			1	
	1	2	8			4	6	
5			4		2		8	7
			2	5	1	9	3	
9	3		7			6		2
	5	8	9	6	3		7	

PUZZLE 13

7		1		5				
9		3	7		6	1		8
	6			3		9		4
2	5		9	8	3	7		
		4		1	5		6	
		9	6	4	7	2	3	5
1		5	3		2			
	3	7		6	1			
		8	5	9	4	3	1	

7		1		5			2	
9		3	7		6	1	5	8
	6			3		9		4
2	5		9	8	3	7		
		4		1	5		6	
		9	6	4	7	2	3	5
1		5	3		2		8	6
	3	7		6	1		9	2
		8	5	9	4	3	1	

2	4				6		8	
		8	2					7
	6		7			4		3
6			8	7		3		1
5		3	1	6	9		4	8
	8	1	3	5	2		7	6
	3	9	4		8	5		2
8	2				3		1	4
1		4	6	2	7	8		9

PUZZLE 16

9		4		8				
3	7	5					1	6
6		2				4	9	3
7		8	6			9	5	
5		3	8		9		2	7
1	4	9	5	7				
		1		2	5	6	8	
			9	3				1
8			4	6	1	2		5

PUZZLE 17

	9	3			6			1
8	4			1	5			
7			3			2	5	
6	3	9	8	7	2		1	5
4			1	3				
	1			5			9	8
1		8	5			6		
9		6			7		4	
	2		9				8	

PUZZLE 18

7	8					5		2
2			7		5		4	
1		5		6	9	7	8	
	1		6	2			5	
4					8	3		6
	5		9	1	3		2	7
9		1			7		6	5
8	7			5	6	9	3	
5		4	3	9				

PUZZLE 19

9		4	1	3				8
7		8				4		
	2				7			
8		1	6	7	9			
				8		9	1	6
					4	5		7
5	7				1		2	
	3		7	9	8			4
4							9	

PUZZLE 20

			1	2		6		
3					4			
		2					1	
4					3		5	
			6					
9				8				4
		3	8	9	5			1
	6					5	7	
			4					8

WORD SEARCH PUZZLES

CHOCOHOLIC

```
C H I P S T R U F F L E S F P
U M A N U A U J O D F J G L R
S N T L S D L R Y D M F L U E
T G F D H H D T M G S I W R T
A H C Y O Z A I E D N S L E Z
R A A B P V V K N D U U E K E
D L D Z Z J E O E G J W T M L
D K B I E L M N O B S W I S S
H N U F U L O H E R S H E Y S
G O R O A R N P B P J I V O C
E U Y P E A N U T R A T Y T O
S B E L G I A N T M U E D D C
E V B S U G A R N S I N I A O
G O D I V A C A K E I N P R A
T F M C A R A M E L Q P T K D
```

Almonds	Belgian	Cadbury	Cake
Caramel	Chips	Cocoa	Custard
Dark	Dove	Godiva	Hazelnuts
Hersheys	Lindt	Milk	Mint
Nuts	Peanut	Pretzels	Pudding
Salted	Shake	Sugar	Sweet
Swiss	Toblerone	Truffles	White

COUNTRIES

```
T O B A G O B U R U N D I J O
A Z E R B A I J A N S R P H U
N K I R I B A T I E B M T T O
Z E N Z P N E B V B O O A G A
A Y B K A R A I S R S U O I A
N P E T I H D U J E N T S R T
I Y U A T L I E L A I Y R N A
A H Z D A T P G V L A O I A J
B W O M I I U H O L D N V M I
F G B R C M L V A N E T N I K
R E U N I O N M A B L M O B I
T A I S E Y C H E L L E S I S
M R C C U D J I B O U T I A T
P S U R I N A M E H T O N G A
C O M O R O S V M A L A W I N
```

Andorra	Azerbaijan	Benin	Bhutan
Bosnia	Burundi	Comoros	Djibouti
Godthab	Kiribati	Lesotho	Malawi
Malaysia	Maldives	Mauritius	Namibia
Principe	Reunion	Seychelles	Suriname
Tajikistan	Tanzania	Tobago	Togo
Tonga	Tuvalu	Vanuatu	Zaire

DICKENS

```
N P C O P P E R F I E L D S P
I M I E B E N E Z E R D Y Y H
C F E R S N O D G R A S S J I
K H S C R O O G E X Y N S Q L
L Y T C H I J N B U M B L E I
E J I R M Z P A D O D G E R P
B G N A J E N N Y W R E N F S
Y D Y T D P I C K W I C K A U
O O T C Y T C Y B V G T I G B
L R I H S C H U Z Z L E W I T
I R M I M D O M B E Y B R N B
V I W T J P L X U M A R L E Y
E T P W I M A G Y R U D G E J
R J D P O R S U D A W K I N S
H A V I S H A M B O F F I N U
```

Boffin	Bumble	Chuzzlewit	Copperfield
Cratchit	Dawkins	Dodger	Dombey
Dorrit	Ebenezer	Fagin	Havisham
Heep	Jenny Wren	Marley	Nancy
Nicholas	Nickleby	Oliver	Philip
Pickwick	Pip	Pirrip	Rudge
Scrooge	Snodgrass	Tiny Tim	Twist

DOGS

```
P O O D L E G R E Y H O U N D
K B A S S E T L T E R R I E R
D O B E R M A N L C O L L I E
P R R E U D A A W H I P P E T
M Z X G E I D R M A S T I F F
X O D R T S E V E C O R G I Z
B I I A E K S P R I N G E R N
I A S D C E R S H E E P D O G
B L Y O L H O F O X H O U N D
A L C G D T S P A N I E L D V
C Z A W O L F H O U N D F I N
O E U S C H N A U Z E R O N L
B S G P O M E R A N I A N G O
D A L M A T I A N N D X N O I
N A C H I H U A H U A C H O W
```

Airedale	Alsatian	Basset	Beagle
Borzoi	Boxer	Chihuahua	Chow
Clydesdale	Cocker	Collie	Corgi
Dachshund	Dalmatian	Dingo	Doberman
Foxhound	Greyhound	Mastiff	Pomeranian
Poodle	Schnauzer	Sheepdog	Spaniel
Springer	Terrier	Whippet	Wolfhound

ANATOMY

```
A N K L E K U Z U R B J W Z T
W I N D P I P E E L B O W O R
L T X V G H T E D T H R O A T
U H O V Y G E I Q W G F M F D
N E C K S T O M A C H K A T B
G M Z A R R S K D Y N V N U L
S J Z E Y K Z Z I I Q I D W A
K D V H S A Y H A V O H I R D
B I T N S R X R P J M E B I D
L O D Z O M B E H U R A L S E
T A N N F S L R R B G R E T R
H Y R E E C E D A X U T G I L
I B X Y S Y R B G T O N G U E
G D O U N A C K M F I N G E R
H P M O E X E P I D E R M I S
```

Ankle	Arms	Bladder	Bones
Brain	Diaphragm	Eardrum	Elbow
Epidermis	Finger	Foot	Heart
Joint	Kidney	Larynx	Liver
Lungs	Mandible	Muscle	Neck
Nose	Stomach	Thigh	Throat
Thyroid	Tongue	Windpipe	Wrist

ARCHITECTURE

```
T R A N S O M B U T T R E S S
E T B A L U S T R A D E L P Y
G O M T W V E N T Y G N L L U
Y W O L U Y L V R T R R I I T
P E D A S T A L I U E T P N R
T R I N C K B T G S C M T T E
I X K T A E U R L C I G I H F
A U C E N Y T E Y A A A C L O
N E O S T S M F P N N R A A I
L S R T I T E O H M E G L R L
A H N D L O N I U T A O L C A
N A I O E N T L U R P Y M H R
C F C R V E O L T U H L N Z C
E T H I E C O S C O X E O I H
T Z E C R V A P I L L A R A A
```

Abutment	Arch	Astragal	Atlantes
Balustrade	Buttress	Cantilever	Column
Corniche	Cupola	Doric	Egyptian
Elliptical	Gargoyle	Grecian	Keystone
Lancet	Pedastal	Pillar	Plinth
Shaft	Tower	Transom	Trefoil
Trefoil Arch	Triglyph	Tuscan	Volute

ELEMENTS, MY DEAR WATSON

```
N I C K E L R A D I U M N X A
C P L U T O N I U M L O U D E
C O L U R A N I U M B N L C U
A I P A F F H Z X R R O S H Z
L B H P T N R G A B G P R R Z
C A M E E I Y C E E S A S O I
I R H Q L R N N W R G R C M N
U I X A U I I U E Y L S O I C
M U R C P R U V M L J E B U R
O M R K O L L M N L S N A M C
T E L L B I J O A I S I L D I
M Z H P S T D S N U Y C T E R
W C A R P A A L U M I N U M O
N H Y D R O G E N O X Y G E N
K R Y P T O N S E L E N I U M
```

Aluminum	Arsenic	Barium	Beryllium
Boron	Calcium	Carbon	Chlorine
Chromium	Cobalt	Copper	Gold
Helium	Hydrogen	Iron	Krypton
Lead	Mercury	Nickel	Oxygen
Platinum	Plutonium	Radium	Radon
Selenium	Silver	Uranium	Zinc

DEITIES

```
B A C C H U S N E P T U N E A
R R O A P O S E I D O N Q R G
I T N B J X O N B K M E O B B
P E C R O N O S I X W L A L F
N M O R P H E U S K F C D G O
X I A N U B I S R U E S I E R
A S T A R T E E A P R L S N T
A U F Z D F T P Y A A A C I U
P L U T O I A B M Q P C O U N
C H Q C P M A U A Y O E R S A
U C W U H L T N N A L R D M L
P M J A L I L C A A L E I L S
I K R I S H N A M D O S A E L
D B G W M E R C U R Y U R C D
M I N E R V A O H E R A I A D
```

Anubis	Apollo	Ares	Artemis
Astarte	Baal	Bacchus	Brahma
Ceres	Cronos	Cupid	Diana
Discordia	Fauna	Flora	Fortuna
Genius	Hera	Jupiter	Krishna
Mars	Mercury	Minerva	Morpheus
Neptune	Nike	Pluto	Poseidon

RIVERS

```
K A G E R A C L H T K N R X M
A M A Z O N O I I A E L P A R
S I Y M A M R P L M V D G I J
A R K A N S A S I B P L U J E
I Y U G G C N W N O O Q A G F
M A C D R H G N D V N N P C F
I N O A U E I U Q H J O Q E
S G L L N R V G S S J R R L R
S T U E D C B E I G C L Q O S
O Z M N E H L R Y U K O N R O
U E B A P I K Y E L L O W A N
R G I U N L O G H Z I B M D O
I S A D R L T I G R I S I O H
R I O G R A N D E S N A K E I
M E K O N G L B U L N G B K O
```

Amazon	Arkansas	Churchill	Colorado
Columbia	Grande	Indus	Jefferson
Kagera	Kasai	Krishna	Limpopo
Magdalena	Mekong	Missouri	Niger
Nile	Ohio	Orange	Rio Grande
Snake	Tambo	Tigris	Ural
Volga	Yangtze	Yellow	Yukon

71

MONEY AND FINANCE

```
P E N S I O N A C C R U E S S
O S I N V E S T M E N T D K J
E E A T A V E R A G I N G Z V
A C P K C H C M N X O D C E O
C U P O N E R T B E F E E S
C R R A P A S S E T S S B N X
U I A I E T B D K I A C I
M T E Y R A N C R I Y L R N
U Y S R E G B I F Y A T A A U
L O E T E A N W T O T N N T M
A D N R B O O K S S C T C E B
T I G Z T H N H U O P B E H E
E G L K C H A R G E S L A L R
A C C O U N T I N G T V U N M
M I N U S D E B I T M P E S K
```

Accounting	Accrue	Accumulate	Aggregate
Appraise	Assets	Averaging	Balance
Bank	Bonds	Books	Branch
Charges	Credit	Debit	Fees
Interest	Investment	Minus	Number
Payee	Payer	Pension	Plus
Rate	Security	Taxes	Trust

CAPITALS

```
R I U D B O G O T A Y F R Y P
O C B E R N K B E R L I N W R
M A D R I D B U D A P E S T E
E N K J A Q Z F M O S C O W T
R B I P A R I S A T O K Y O O
Q E V A M S T E R D A M S L R
B R Y O T T A W A Z O G T O I
D R T K F V D U B L I N O N A
C A L N J H O I S Y U D C D T
V I E N N A M O N A C O K O N
H A V A N A V L I M A D H N S
A T H E N S V I R H P I O Y E
H E L S I N K I K M F E L G O
B R U S S E L S B M K D M O U
Y K V W M F S A N T I A G O L
```

Amsterdam	Athens	Beijing	Berlin
Bern	Bogota	Brussels	Budapest
Canberra	Dublin	Havana	Helsinki
Lima	London	Madrid	Monaco
Moscow	Oslo	Ottawa	Paris
Pretoria	Reykjavik	Rome	Santiago
Seoul	Stockholm	Tokyo	Vienna

CLOTHES

```
C A R D I G A N C B L O U S E
C A F T A N T Y G B T C O A T
L C M K W E F N T L I H U T N
O R T Q K I W B E Y O B L I D
A A J C B O B B E A H V K I I
K I A R G E L B A R R R E Z C
C J L R S V A B V T E C B S Q
B Z O N J F Z N I J H T T I B
K I A M B E E J I K R R W I S
Y E F I A V R T F E I S O T C
J T E T P T G S L F S N O B V
G L R T R R A W E E Z O I V E
E O S E O M O A R Y B H Z P U
X V E N N B T D M S N B A H A
J H Z S L I P P E R S C L O G
```

Apron	Arctic	Bathrobe	Beanie
Belt	Beret	Bib	Bikini
Blazer	Blouse	Boots	Bowler
Caftan	Cape	Cardigan	Cloak
Clog	Coat	Dress	Gloves
Gown	Jacket	Jeans	Jerkin
Jersey	Loafers	Mittens	Slippers

SHAKESPEARE

```
H A M L E T M E R C H A N T C
E N G L I S H N T E M P E S T
C J S V C O M E D Y S H R E W
W L U P L A Y W R I G H T K L
I I E L P E R I C L E S C H C
T M L O I A N D G T I M O N Y
C M R L P E N Z R W O U R Y M
H M D T I A T T O A S A I U B
E A V O N A T E O U M T O T E
S C B W T D M R T N U A L R L
P B A N O O Z I A C Y C A A I
Q E S T R A T F O R D L N G N
O T H E L L O D N H Z E U E E
O H K X E P L A Y M V A S D V
E R R O R S R I C H A R D Y J
```

Antony	Avon	Cleopatra	Comedy
Coriolanus	Cymbeline	Drama	English
Errors	Hamlet	Juliet	Lear
Macbeth	Merchant	Othello	Pericles
Play	Playwright	Richard	Romeo
Shrew	Stratford	Tempest	Timon
Titus	Tragedy	William	Witches

IT'S THE LAW

```
C P H D D E M U R R E R O B R
R C S W I P V F X S V R C A D
I U E K Z S F E U N I A B N D
M Q N W C I C A R A C A S E I
I L T X L D C L B D T Z Q T S
N E E E V G E V A S I V E S S
A G N Z B J A W Q I M C E W E
L A C A V E A T I A M F T G N
P C E B E Q U E S T I E D D T
A Y O P I N I O N A N U R X L
I N J U N C T I O N J E K U A
E S S E N T I A L B U U S B L
C O V E R T S I D E B A R S I
E V I D E N C E B E N C H Y B
D A M A G E S L A W S U I T I
```

Alibi	Bar	Bench	Bequest
Case	Cause	Caveat	Covert
Criminal	Damages	Demurrer	Disclaimer
Dissent	Essential	Evasive	Evidence
Injunction	Judge	Jury	Lawsuit
Legacy	Opinion	Panel	Sentence
Sidebar	Verdict	Victim	Witness

CHEMISTRY

```
A L C O H O L A T B O H R C B
B B B T A C C E L E R A T O R
S I R C I O B C P K E S N B O
O S O A W N R D M S A H T A N
R M M R V D M U A F C L A L Z
P U I B A U I B A Y T M O T E
T T D O A C V Z O N I N N I K
I H E N L T I A M M O N I A D
O O R A Z O T D B O N D T W A
N O C B C R B E I N M B E A L
C D Q W X M U E R T Z U F T C
N X A A F G I R R Y Y N A T H
C O R R O S I O N Y U S T J E
V O C A F F E I N E L E O V M
B E S S E M E R O H F N M O Y
```

Absorption	Accelerator	Acidity	Alchemy
Alcohol	Alkaloid	Ammonia	Anode
Atom	Base	Battery	Beryl
Bessemer	Bismuth	Bohr	Bond
Borax	Bromide	Bronze	Bunsen
Caffeine	Calcium	Carbon	Cobalt
Conductor	Corrosion	Reaction	Watt

WHAT GOES UP, MUST COME DOWN (PHYSICS)

```
S T R A I N K U N I V E R S E
S P E C T R U M P H O T O N I
V E L P O T E N T I A L I P S
Q U A W R A D I A T I O N O O
D M T U N D U L A T I O N W L
O F I P V W L M S O L I D E A
S S V I B R A T I O N D U R R
U P I P E T F N W P H A R Y N
P A T V R A S M A U Q O I O W
E C Y O E O U T R L T U I V A
R E G L A U T C R S O S A G V
N T V T C C J O I E R G A R E
O I O A T T Q S N O S N I G K
V M V G O D E C T E N S I O N
A E X E R R O O W S T E R E O
```

Analog	Photon	Potential	Power
Proton	Pulse	Quark	Radiation
Reactor	Relativity	Resistor	Solar
Solid	Spacetime	Spectrum	Stereo
Strain	Stress	Supernova	Tension
Torsion	Undulation	Universe	Vacuum
Vibration	Voltage	Wave	Work

COMPOSERS

```
S O N D H E I M T O M K I N S
Z W I L I C H U C O W A R D W
S H O S T A K O V I C H R V H
B A P T C S T R O Z Z I F I I
J R A C H M A N I N O V W V T
V B H P A O I T V K O G E A E
V E R D I Z M K O K I F B L M
S R V T K A C P A R D N E D A
C N I H O R W S S X E P R I N
H S P A V T R T C O P L A N D
U T S L S O V A X V N U L D Q
B E O B K W I L L I A M S I B
E I U E Y X H L Y V E L G A R
R N S R O D R I G O S E N F L
T W A G N E R S A L I E R I V
```

Bernstein	Copland	Coward	Elgar
Korsakov	Mozart	Rachmaninov	Rodrigo
Salieri	Schubert	Senfl	Shostakovich
Sondheim	Sousa	Strozzi	Tallis
Tchaikovsky	Thalberg	Thompson	Tomkins
Torelli	Verdi	Vivaldi	Wagner
Weber	Whiteman	Williams	Zwilich

MUSHROOMS

```
E  R  I  N  G  I  K  I  T  R  U  F  F  L  E
N  I  T  F  M  Y  G  O  L  D  E  N  R  S  M
B  C  U  A  A  A  P  Y  T  L  Q  R  L  U  A
P  U  A  T  B  L  I  S  G  I  R  E  S  X  T
P  U  T  R  B  L  S  T  Y  P  R  D  H  C  S
S  P  F  T  D  E  E  E  A  O  W  P  I  T  U
P  J  C  F  O  O  W  R  M  K  L  I  T  X  T
U  H  X  J  B  N  N  I  U  B  E  N  A  W  A
B  L  A  C  K  A  J  C  N  P  R  E  K  O  K
R  E  I  S  H  I  L  Y  E  T  S  O  E  L  E
C  R  I  M  I  N  I  L  Z  L  E  T  W  F  Z
B  U  R  G  U  N  D  Y  A  E  L  R  R  N  H
C  H  A  N  T  E  R  E  L  L  E  O  U  A  Y
P  A  R  A  S  O  L  T  R  U  M  P  E  T  W
H  E  D  G  E  H  O  G  O  C  B  E  E  C  H
```

Beech	Black	Brown	Burgundy
Button	Cardoncello	Chanterelle	Crimini
Eringi	False	Golden	Gypsy
Hedgehog	Maitake	Matsutake	Morels
Oyster	Parasol	Puffball	Red Pine
Reishi	Shitake	Straw	Table
Truffle	Trumpet	Winter	Wolf

TREES AND SHRUBS

```
B S M P F Y O D V M A Z N C Q
W P A C A J P M V M A O F I R
A R G H M P E S A Q M N H W E
L U N E W C A D W E X C G O J
N C O S I I C W L O R F L O Z
U E L T Z J H N F I L A A Y L
T E I N P I N E B M O I O E M
N U A U N S E Q U O I A V W I
P W L T M C R L A U R E L E M
E I P I N E P O A V O C A D O
C L Q E P T I G E R W O O D S
A L D L P M A H O G A N Y P A
N O W A J P U L L Y H I N E E
Y W P I I R E D W O O D H A J
S T R A W B E R R Y H F C R B
```

Aloe	Avocado	Birch	Chestnut
Fir	Laurel	Lemon	Magnolia
Mahogany	Mango	Mimosa	Olive
Papaw	Peach	Pear	Pecan
Pepper	Pine	Plum	Redwood
Sequoia	Spruce	Strawberry	Tigerwood
Tulip	Walnut	Willow	Yew

HANDSOME ACTORS WE'VE SEEN

```
R M C Q U E E N K E W B C Y P
E A J R L W E S G P A K E S Y
D R M E E A A E G X C N V K T
F T Z Y G S S K Y G O B T A B
O I G N E H T B L O D J W R R
R N R O N I W E L S E G I S A
D X A L D N O C E L A J L G N
I M N D O G O K N I N N L A D
S C T S E T D F H N W E I R O
H I D T M O Y O A G G W A D Q
E U T O I N E R A K L M M E M
H I O R G M N D L X O A S M R
P L H P R E S L E Y V N A Q C
B T I M B E R L A K E H S K H
S T A M O S W E R F R J C I O
```

Beckford	Bloom	Brando	Cho
Clooney	Dean	Eastwood	Gere
Glover	Gosling	Grant	Gyllenhaal
Hamm	Hudson	Legend	Llenhaal
Martin	Mcqueen	Newman	Pitt
Presley	Redford	Reynolds	Skarsgard
Stamos	Timberlake	Washington	Williams

WORD JUMBLES

PUZZLE 1

"Anyone who believes what a _____ deserves all he gets."

- Neil Gaiman

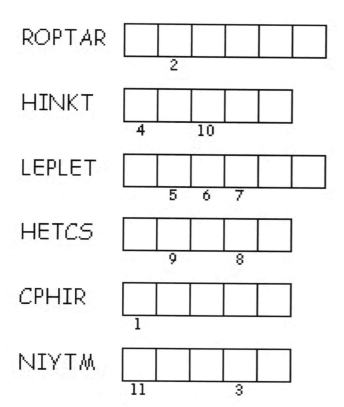

ROPTAR

HINKT

LEPLET

HETCS

CPHIR

NIYTM

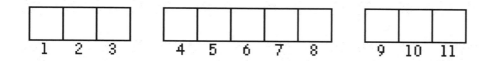

PUZZLE 2

"Dogs come when they're called; cats take a message and get
_____."

- Mary Bly

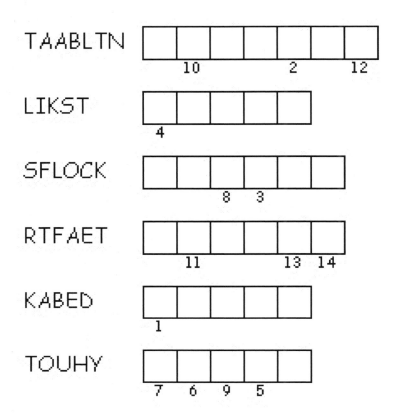

TAABLTN

LIKST

SFLOCK

RTFAET

KABED

TOUHY

PUZZLE 3

"Humans: No fur, no paws, no tail. They run away from mice.
They never get enough sleep. How can you help but love such an
_____?"

- Anonymous Cat

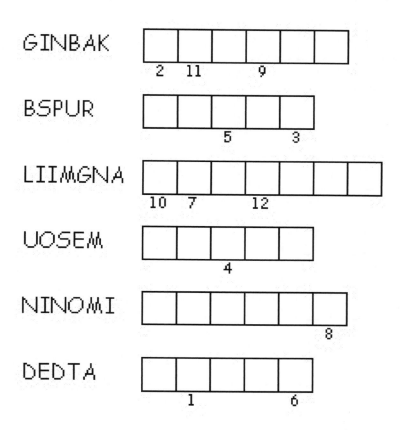

GINBAK

BSPUR

LIIMGNA

UOSEM

NINOMI

DEDTA

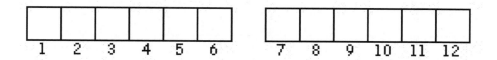

PUZZLE 4

"If a black cat crosses your path, it signifies that the animal is

_____

- Groucho Marx

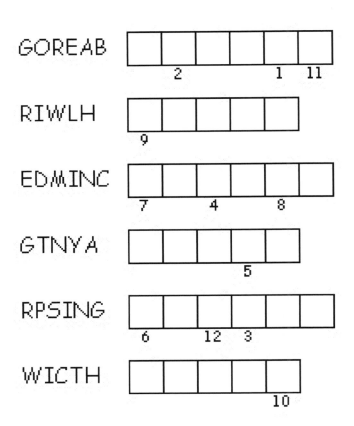

GOREAB

	2			1	11

RIWLH

9				

EDMINC

7		4		8	

GTNYA

			5	

RPSING

6		12	3		

WICTH

				10

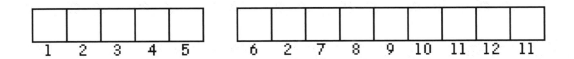

1	2	3	4	5

6	2	7	8	9	10	11	12	11

PUZZLE 5

"There is nothing noble in being superior to your fellow man; true nobility is being superior to _____."

- Ernest Hemmingway

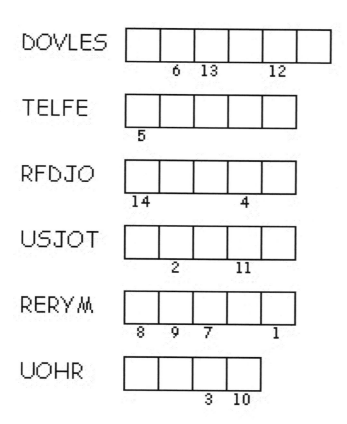

DOVLES `___ ___ ___ ___ ___ ___`
        6   13   12

TELFE `___ ___ ___ ___ ___`
       5

RFDJO `___ ___ ___ ___ ___`
       14   4

USJOT `___ ___ ___ ___ ___`
            2   11

RERYM `___ ___ ___ ___ ___`
       8   9   7   1

UOHR `___ ___ ___ ___`
           3   10

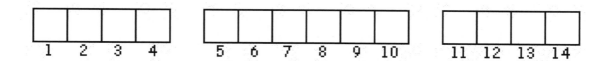

| 1 | 2 | 3 | 4 | | 5 | 6 | 7 | 8 | 9 | 10 | | 11 | 12 | 13 | 14 |

PUZZLE 6

"Whether you believe you can do a thing or not, _____. "

- Henry Ford

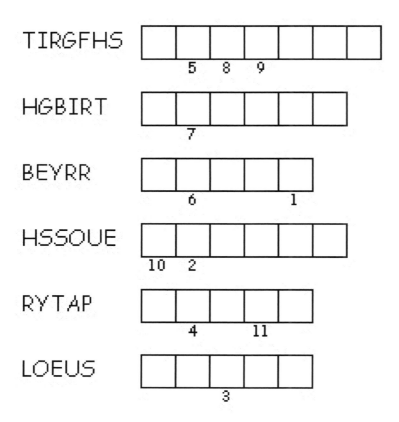

TIRGFHS

⬜⬜⬜⬜⬜⬜⬜
    5   8   9

HGBIRT

⬜⬜⬜⬜⬜⬜
    7

BEYRR

⬜⬜⬜⬜⬜
   6   1

HSSOUE

⬜⬜⬜⬜⬜⬜
10 2

RYTAP

⬜⬜⬜⬜⬜
   4   11

LOEUS

⬜⬜⬜⬜⬜
   3

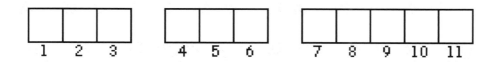

⬜⬜⬜ ⬜⬜⬜ ⬜⬜⬜⬜⬜
1 2 3   4 5 6   7 8 9 10 11

PUZZLE 7

"Some men see things as they are and ask why. Others dream things that never were and _____."

- George Bernard Shaw

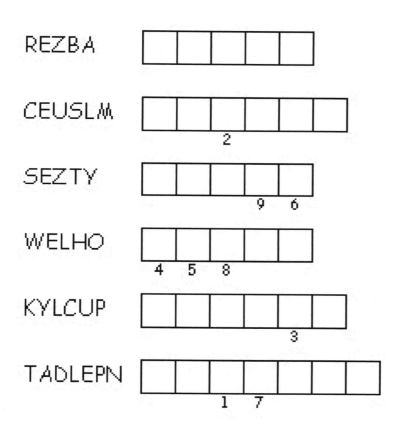

REZBA

CEUSLM
2

SEZTY
9 6

WELHO
4 5 8

KYLCUP
3

TADLEPN
1 7

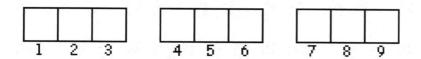
1 2 3   4 5 6   7 8 9

PUZZLE 8

I like pigs. Dogs look up to us. Cats look down on us. Pigs

_____.

- Winston Churchill

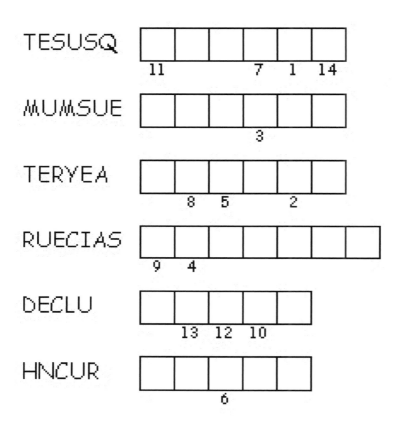

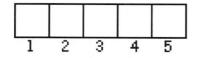 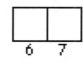 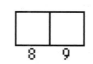 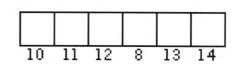

90

PUZZLE 9

"Never memorize something that _____."

- Albert Einstein

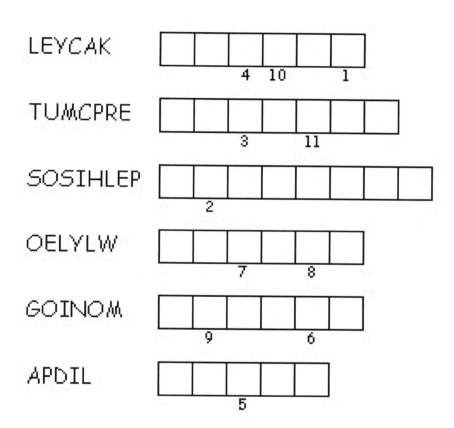

LEYCAK

			4	10		1

TUMCPRE

		3		11		

SOSIHLEP

OELYLW

GOINOM

APDIL

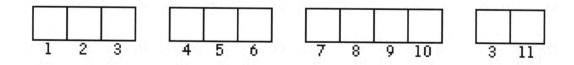

PUZZLE 10

"Get your facts first, and then you _____ as much as you please. "

- Mark Twain

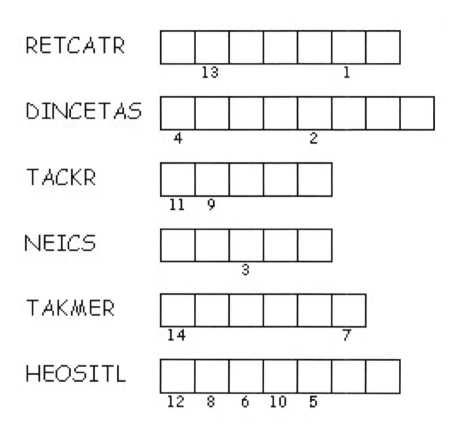

RETCATR

DINCETAS

TACKR

NEICS

TAKMER

HEOSITL

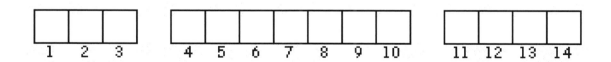

PUZZLE 11

"Always forgive your enemies; _____ so much."

- Oscar Wilde

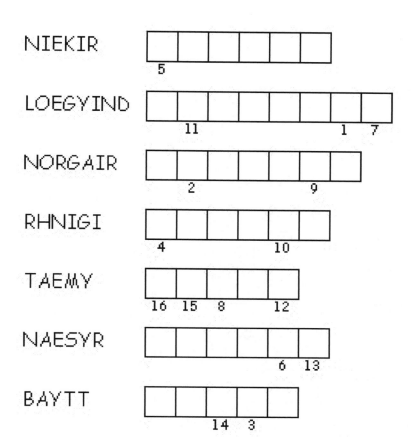

NIEKIR

LOEGYIND

NORGAIR

RHNIGI

TAEMY

NAESYR

BAYTT

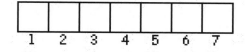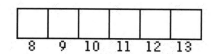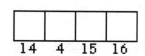

PUZZLE 12

"A lie gets halfway around the world before the truth has a chance to _____."

- Winston Churchill

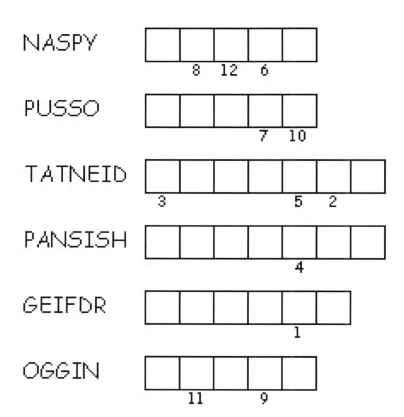

NASPY

PUSSO

TATNEID

PANSISH

GEIFDR

OGGIN

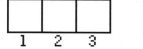 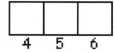 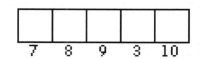 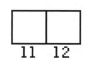

PUZZLE 13

"I like long walks, especially when they are taken by people

_____."

- Fred Allen

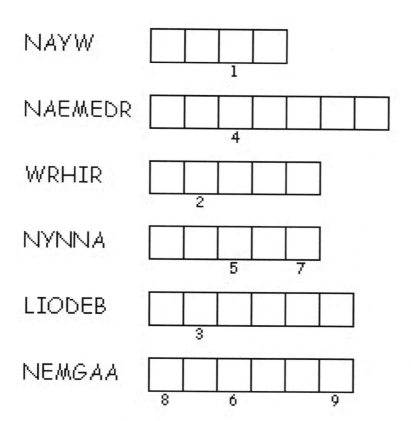

NAYW

NAEMEDR

WRHIR

NYNNA

LIODEB

NEMGAA

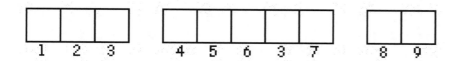

PUZZLE 14

"I'm not crazy about reality, but it's still the only place to get
_____."

- Groucho Marx

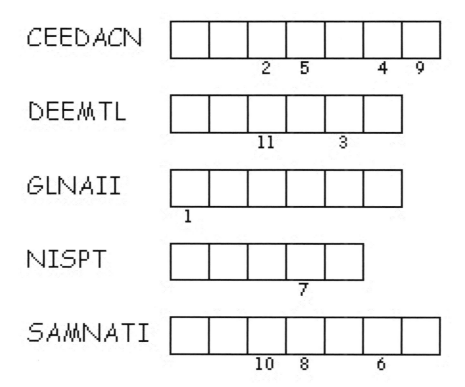

CEEDACN

DEEMTL

GLNAII

NISPT

SAMNATI

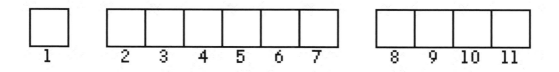

PUZZLE 15

"Never put off till tomorrow what may be done _____ just as well."

- Mark Twain

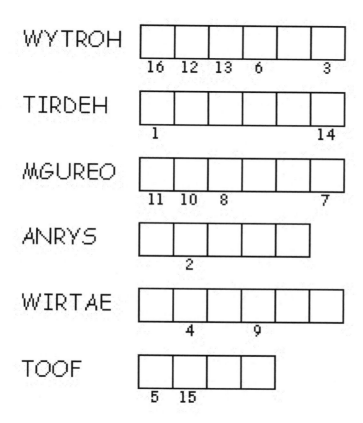

WYTROH

16	12	13	6		3

TIRDEH

1					14

MGUREO

11	10	8			7

ANRYS

	2			

WIRTAE

	4		9		

TOOF

5	15		

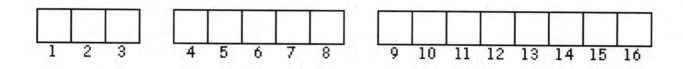

1	2	3

4	5	6	7	8

9	10	11	12	13	14	15	16

PUZZLE 16

"I _____. I love the whooshing noise they make as they go by."

- Douglas Adams

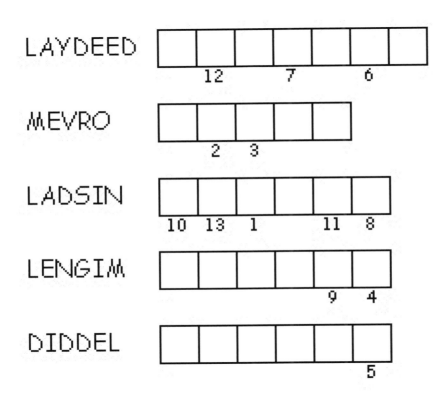

LAYDEED

	12		7		6	

MEVRO

	2	3		

LADSIN

10	13	1		11	8

LENGIM

				9	4

DIDDEL

				5	

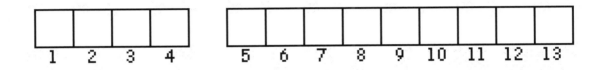

1	2	3	4

5	6	7	8	9	10	11	12	13

PUZZLE 17

"I never travel without _____. One should always have something sensational to read in the train."

- Oscar Wilde

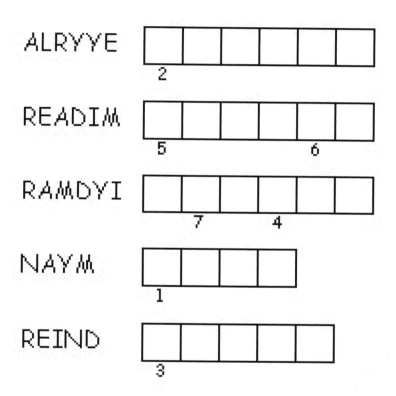

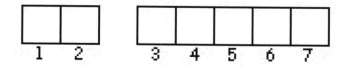

PUZZLE 18

"I'm sure the universe is full of intelligent life. It's just been
_____ to come here."

- Arthur C. Clarke

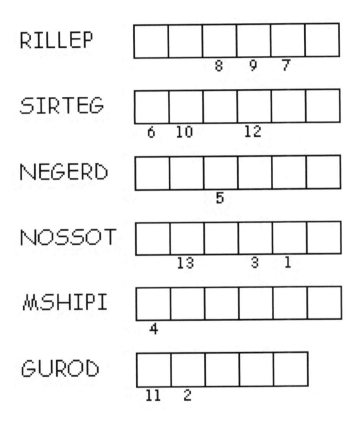

RILLEP

SIRTEG

NEGERD

NOSSOT

MSHIPI

GUROD

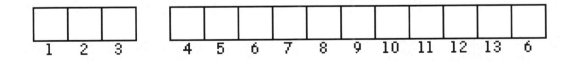

PUZZLE 19

"Outside of a dog, a book is man's best friend. Inside of a dog it's
_____."

- Groucho Marx

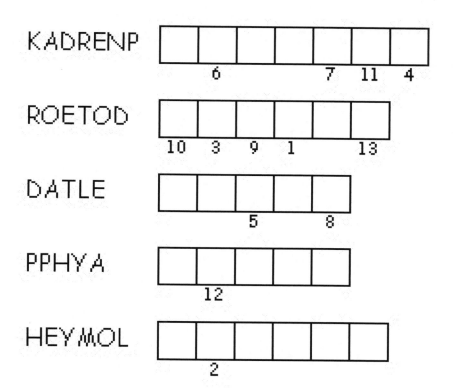

KADRENP ⬜⬜⬜⬜⬜⬜⬜
          6   7 11 4

ROETOD ⬜⬜⬜⬜⬜⬜
       10 3 9 1   13

DATLE ⬜⬜⬜⬜⬜
          5   8

PPHYA ⬜⬜⬜⬜⬜
       12

HEYMOL ⬜⬜⬜⬜⬜
        2

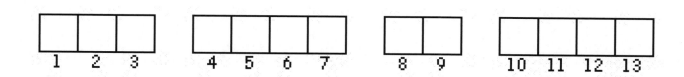

| 1 | 2 | 3 | | 4 | 5 | 6 | 7 | | 8 | 9 | | 10 | 11 | 12 | 13 |

PUZZLE 20

"A boy can learn a lot from a dog: obedience, loyalty, and the importance of turning around three times _____."
- Robert Benchley

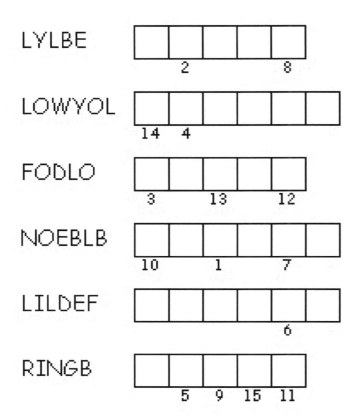

LYLBE

LOWYOL

FODLO

NOEBLB

LILDEF

RINGB

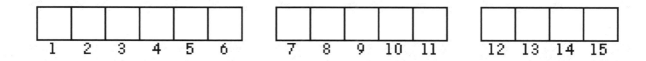

WORD FIT PUZZLES

PUZZLE #1
IN A RECIPE BOOK

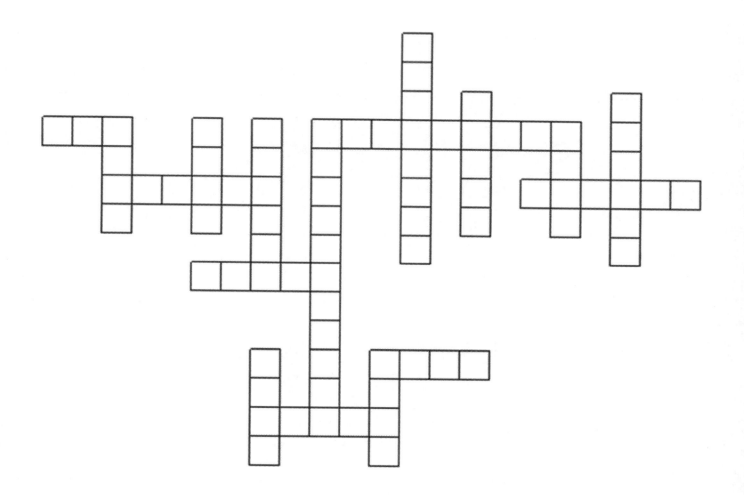

baking   beat   beef   cups

desserts   lamb   metric   oil

pasta   pork   recipe   soups

stews   stir   tablespoons   teaspoons

timing

PUZZLE #2
A RISK OF LOBSTERS?
COLLECTIVE ANIMAL NAMES

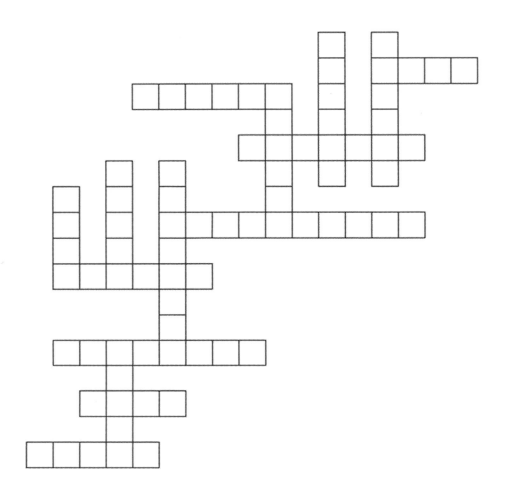

army   business   cackle
cauldron   pack   parade
pounce   prickle   pride
romp   shadow   stand
tower   unkindness   warren

PUZZLE #3
THE ANIMALS IN PUZZLE #2

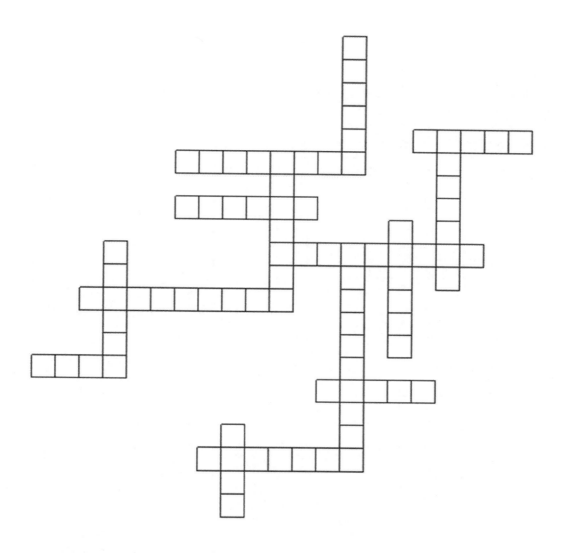

elephants
porcupines
otters
hyenas
lions

ferrets
flamingos
rabbits
frogs
bats

giraffes
ravens
jaguars
wolves
cats

PUZZLE #4
ONE WORD MOVIES

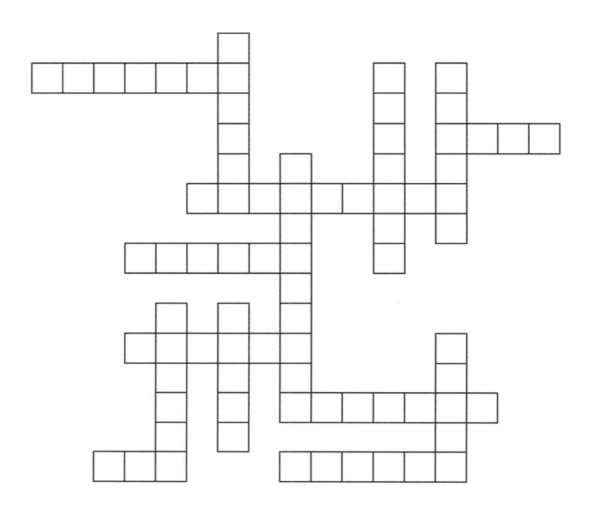

Batman	Casino	Chinatown
Fargo	Hamlet	Lolita
Mash	Nashville	Network
Nixon	Othello	Patton
Psycho	Ran	Vertigo

PUZZLE #5
BOOKS WITH ONE WORD TITLES

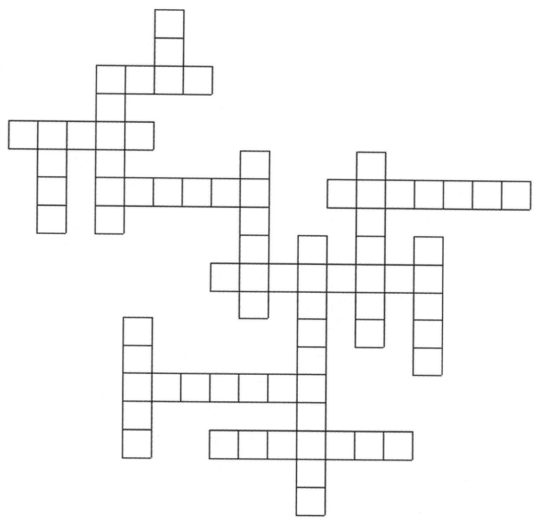

Persuasion

Rebecca

Heidi

Exodus

Kim

Timeline

Candide

Utopia

Babbitt

Proof

Carrie

Matilda

Nerve

Emma

Risk

PUZZLE #6
SONGS FROM THE 1950's

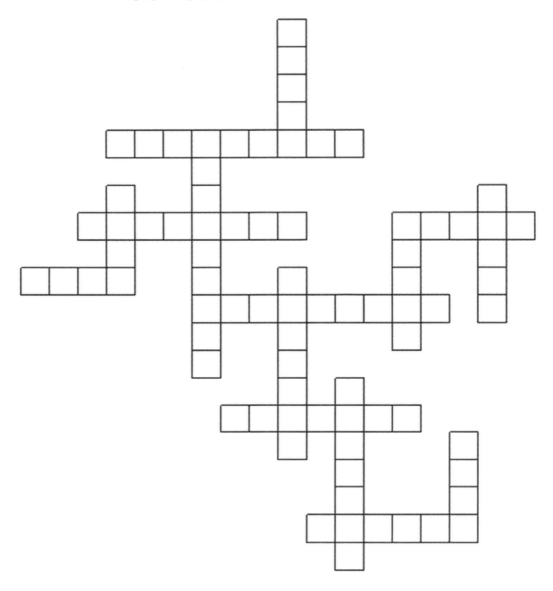

Bewitched   Diana   Gone
Honeycomb   Jambalaya   Jezebel
Lollipop   More   Pretend
Ruby   Slowly   Tammy
Tequila   Tiger   Venus

PUZZLE #7
SONGS FROM THE 1960's

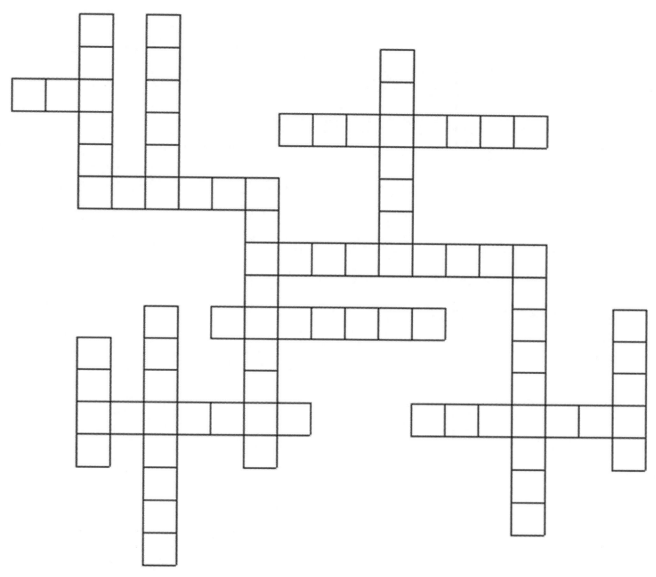

Because
Downtown
One
Runaway
Volare'

Calcutta
Fire
Raindrops
Sherry
Wheels

Cherish
Night
Respect
Surrender
Yesterday

PUZZLE #8
SONGS ABOUT WOMEN

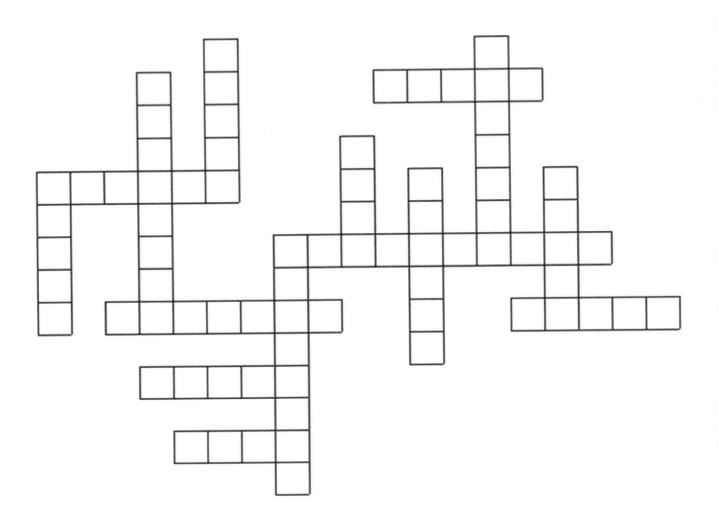

Diana
Jean
Maybellene
Sheila
Tammy

Donna
Jezebel
Patricia
Sherry
Valleri

Honey
Marianne
Ruby
Sunny
Windy

PUZZLE #9
SOME U.S. STATES

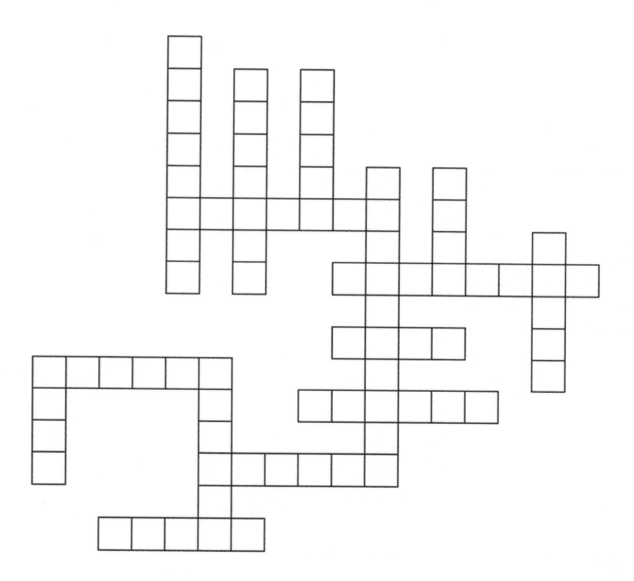

Alaska   Arizona   California
Colorado   Florida   Idaho
Iowa   Kansas   Maine
Michigan   Nevada   Ohio
Oregon   Texas   Utah

PUZZLE #10
THEM BONES

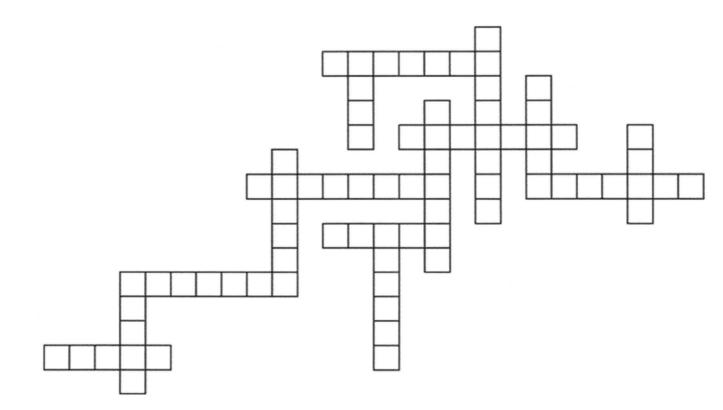

clavicle	frontal	humerus
hyoid	mandible	maxilla
nasal	patella	radius
ribs	sacrum	sternum
talus	tibia	ulna

PUZZLE #11
TV SHOWS IN A WORD

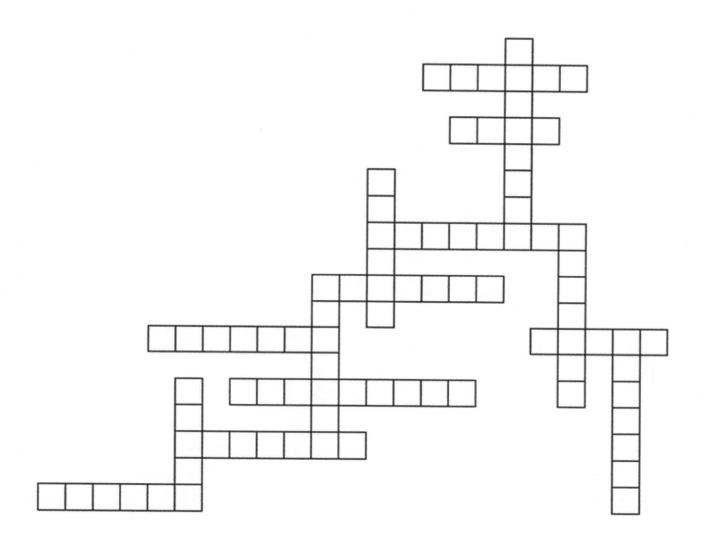

Bewitched
Columbo
Friends
Mash
Scrubs

Bonanza
Dynasty
Gunsmoke
Newhart
Seinfeld

Cheers
Frasier
Lassie
Psych
Wings

PUZZLE #12
SONGS ABOUT MEN

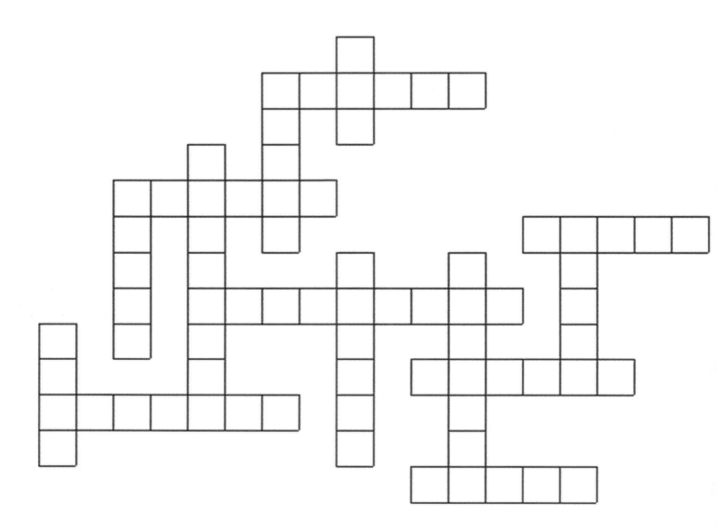

Ahab   Alejandro   Alexis
Alfie   Andrew   Anthony
Atlas   Basil   Ben
Caesar   Craig   Daniel
Fernando   Frankie   Jesse

PUZZLE #13
GREAT CAR NAMES

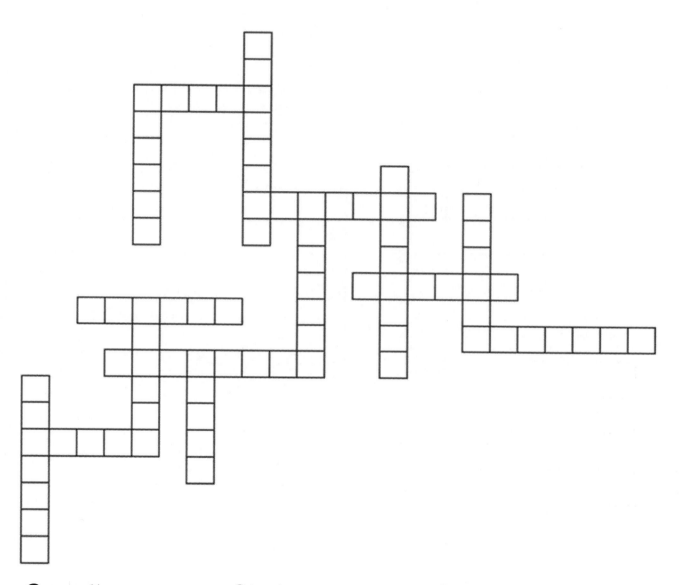

Corvette
Spitfire
Talon
Demon
Diablo

Stratos
Raptor
Legend
Magnum
Mustang

Rampage
Hornet
Vanquish
Viper
Javelin

PUZZLE #14
POPULAR CAT BREEDS

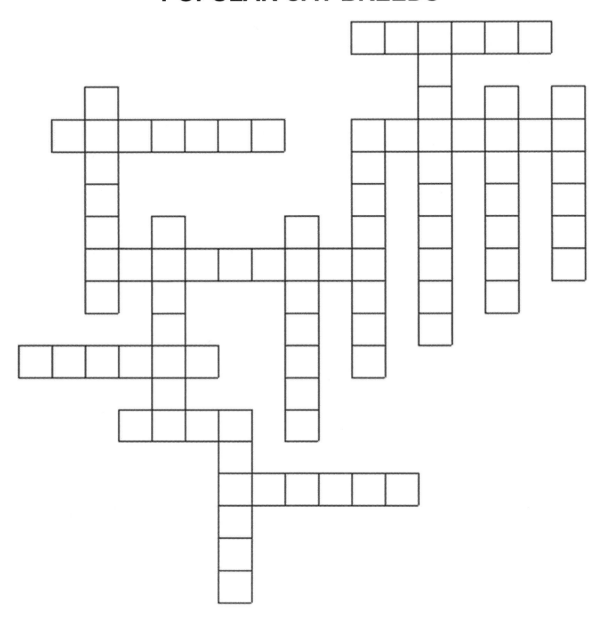

Bengal	Birman	Blue
Bobtail	Bombay	Burmese
Burmese	Exotic	Ocicat
Persian	Ragamuffin	Ragdoll
Shorthair	Siamese	Siberian

PUZZLE #15
SOME CAR PARTS

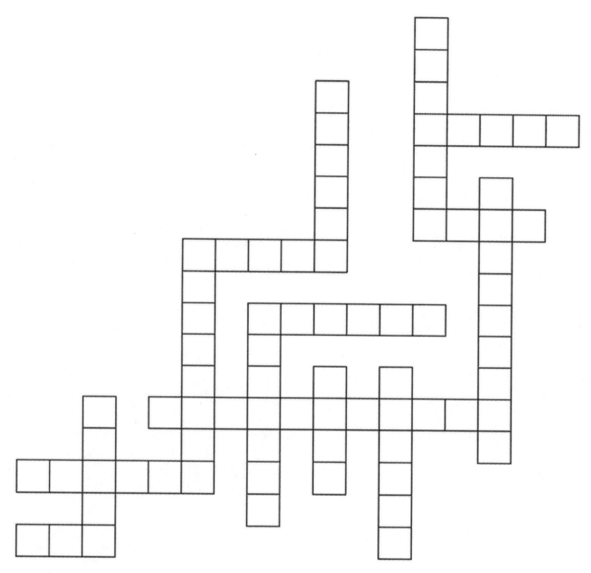

battery	brakes	bumper
dashboard	distributer	doors
engine	gauges	light
mat	rims	seat
tailpipe	tires	windows

PUZZLE #16
15 SHADES OF GREEN

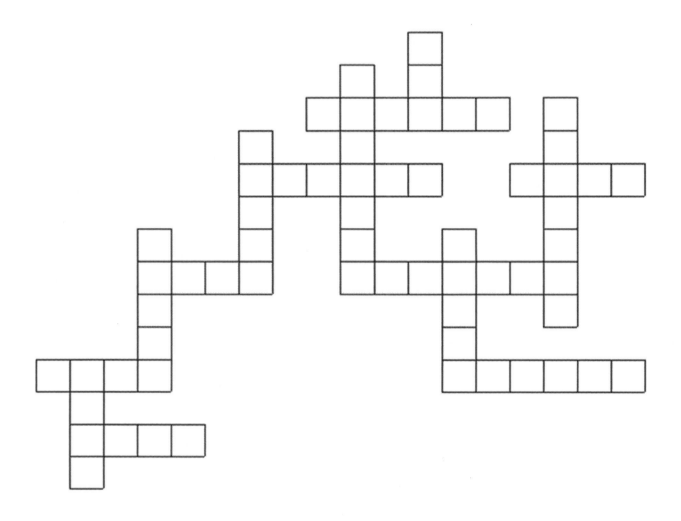

army

grass

lime

olive

spring

avocado

hunter

mint

pasture

tea

emerald

jade

moss

safari

thyme

PUZZLE #17
TV ANIMALS

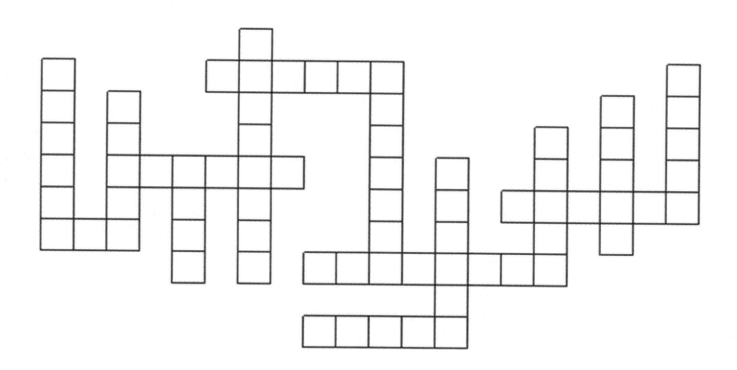

Bandit

Gizmo

Kitty

Salem

Target

Dexter

Grumpy

Lassie

Scratchy

Tom

Garfield

Jerry

Oscar

Spot

Trigger

PUZZLE #18
FIRST LADIES OF THE UNITED STATES

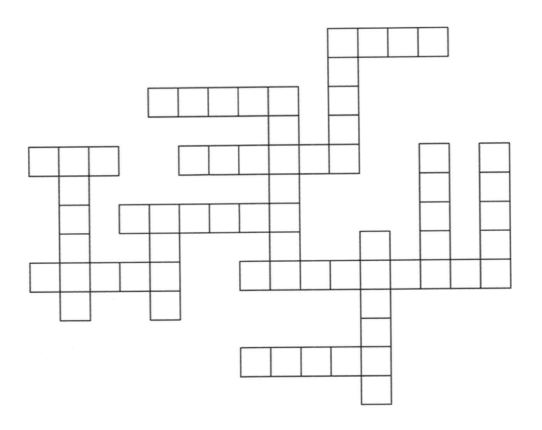

Abigail
Eliza
Helen
Julia
Martha

Anna
Elizabeth
Ida
Louisa
Rachel

Dolley
Grace
Jane
Mamie
Sarah

PUZZLE #19
FLOWER POWER

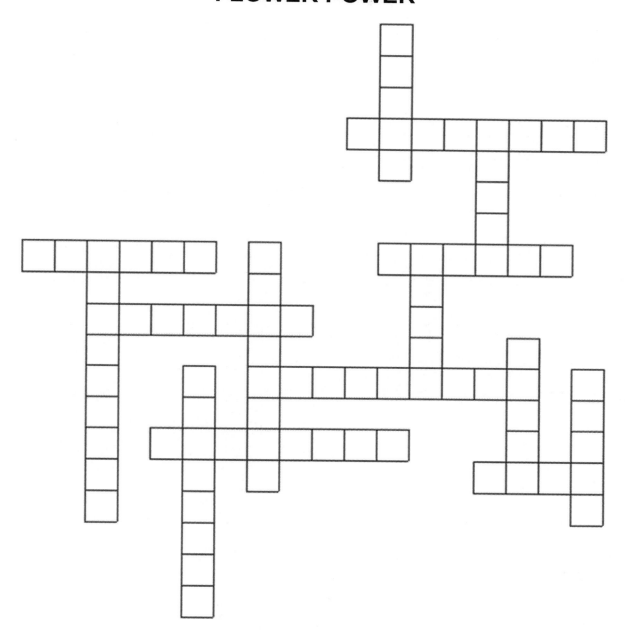

Aster

Dahlia

Hyacinth

Lavender

Oleander

Broom

Daisies

Hydrangea

Lilac

Pansy

Crocus

Foxglove

Iris

Narcissus

Roses

PUZZLE #20
STATIONERY STORE

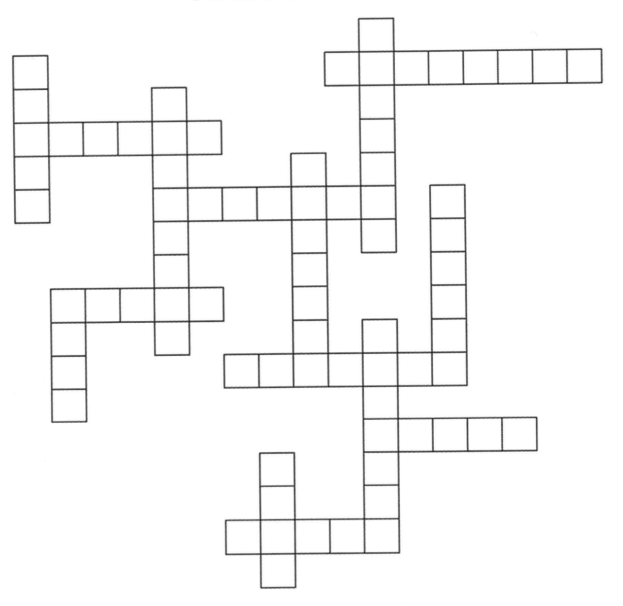

stapler
markers
pencils
boards
tacks

printer
folders
laptop
cards
files

computer
paper
notebook
pens
lead

TOUGH TRIVIA

1. On which island was Napoleon exiled following his defeat at Waterloo?

2. Who was the 'Mad Monk' of Russian history?

3. What is the largest fish in the ocean?

4. What artist painted a mustache and goatee on the Mona Lisa?

5. In which country would one find 8 of the 10 world's highest mountains?

6. Which common word changes its pronunciation when the first letter is capitalized?

7. Which is the only vowel on a standard keyboard not on the top line of letters?

8. What is the longest river in the world?

9. What is the world's tallest mountain (above sea level)?

10. What is the most popular drink in the world that does not contain alcohol?

11. Does sound travel faster through water or steel?

12. What was the first planet to be discovered using a telescope, in 1781?

13. Which country is bordered by both the Atlantic and Indian oceans?

14. What is a group of frogs known as?

15. What is the most common blood type in humans?

16. What is the only word in English ending in the letters 'mt'?

17. Which is the largest known planet in the solar system?

18. What is a group of crows called?

19. What is a group of ravens called?

20. What do you call a group of unicorns?

21. Where was the fortune cookie invented?

22. If cats are feline, and dogs are canine, what are bears?

23. What is paper money made from?

24. Which German city is famous for the perfume it produces?

25. What did the crocodile swallow in Peter Pan?

26. Who did Lady Diana Spencer marry?

27. Where is the smallest bone in the body?

28. Which is the only mammal that can't jump?

29. Who lived at 221B, Baker Street, London?

30. How many dots are there on two dice?

31. Who painted the Mona Lisa?

32. Where does the British Prime Minister live?

33. When did the Second World War end?

34. What are the first three words of the bible?

35. What's the real name of Siddhartha Gautama?

36. What's the name of the famous big clock in London?

37. Where was Christopher Columbus born?

38. When did the American Civil War end?

39. What did the 7 dwarves do for a job?

40. Who painted the Sistine Chapel?

41. Where are the Dolomites?

42. What's the capital of Kenya?

43. Which is the largest ocean?

44. What's the capital of Ethiopia?

45. How many squares are there on a chess board?

46. How many prongs are there on a fork?

47. Who starts first in chess?

48. How many events are there in the decathlon?

49. What language has the most words?

50. What's the Hungarian word for pepper?

51. Name the two main actors in "The Sting".

52. What country gave Florida to the USA in 1891?

53. Who gave his name to the month of July?

54.   What's the most important book in the Moslem religion?

55.   In what decade was Elvis' first ever concert?

56.   Who sang "My Way"?

57.   Who invented the electric light bulb?

58.   What's the smallest type of tree in the world?

59.   What activity other than jumping are kangaroos good at?

60.   What colors make purple?

61.   What's the hardest rock?

62.   Which river goes through London?

SOLUTIONS

CROSSWORDS
SOLUTIONS

PUZZLE #1

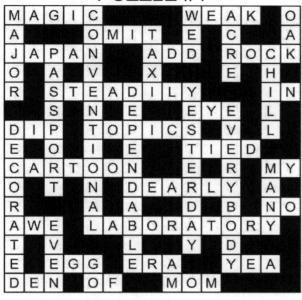

PUZZLE #2

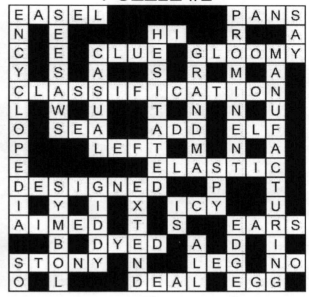

PUZZLE #3

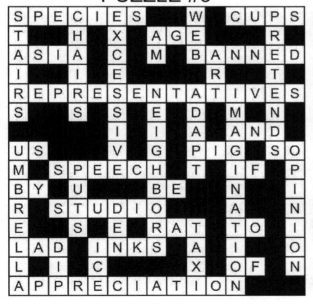

PUZZLE #4

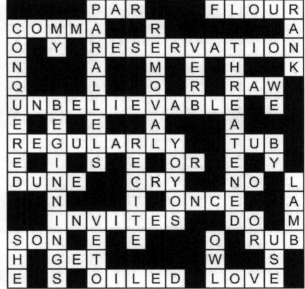

PUZZLE #5

PUZZLE #6

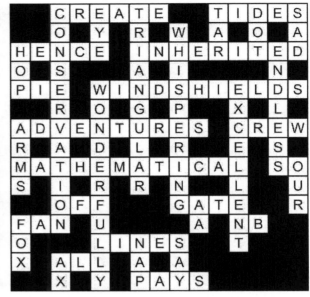

PUZZLE #7

PUZZLE #8

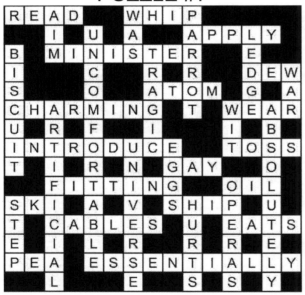

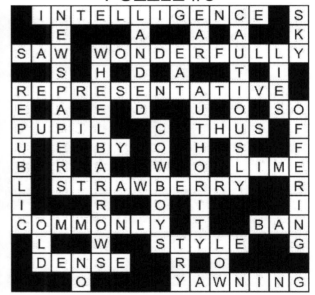

PUZZLE #9

PUZZLE #10

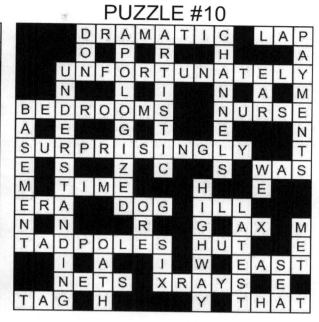

PUZZLE #11

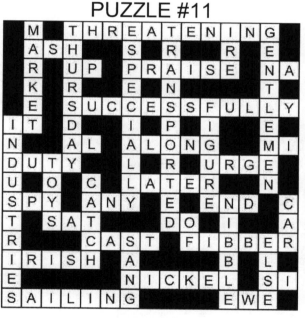

PUZZLE #12

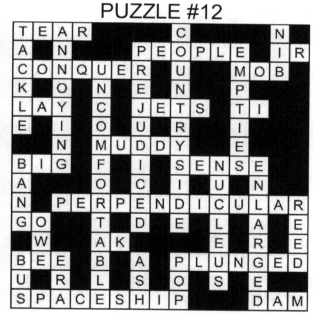

PUZZLE #13

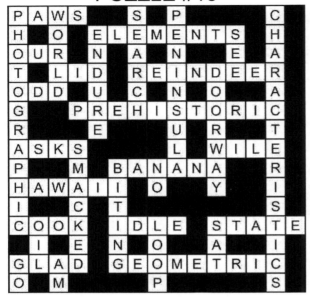

PUZZLE #14

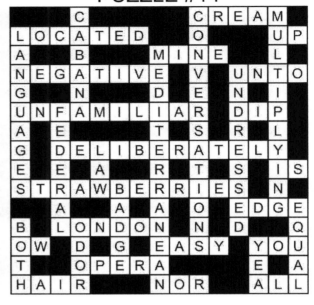

PUZZLE #15

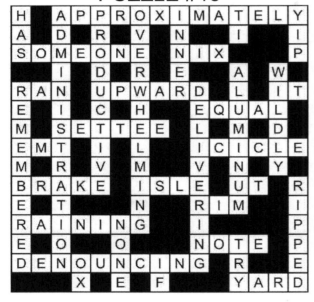

PUZZLE #16

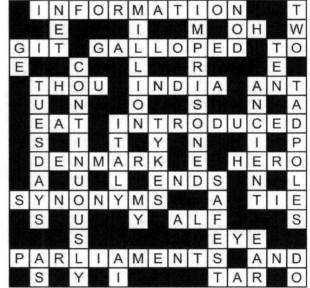

PUZZLE #17

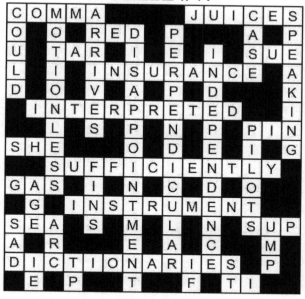

PUZZLE #18

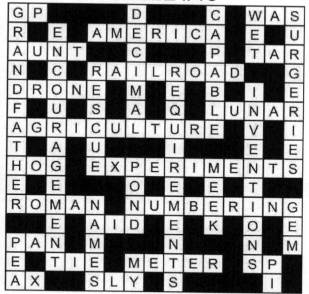

PUZZLE #19

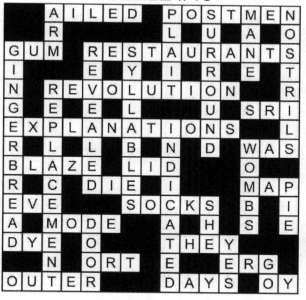

PUZZLE #20

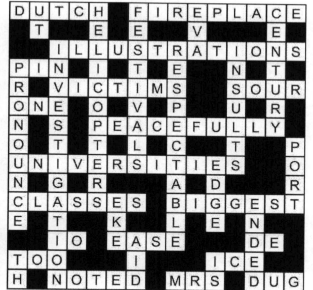

SUDOKU
SOLUTIONS

PUZZLE #1

5	1	6	8	9	2	7	4	3
9	2	7	4	5	3	6	1	8
3	8	4	7	6	1	5	9	2
6	7	1	2	4	9	3	8	5
8	3	9	6	7	5	4	2	1
4	5	2	3	1	8	9	6	7
1	4	3	5	2	6	8	7	9
2	6	8	9	3	7	1	5	4
7	9	5	1	8	4	2	3	6

PUZZLE #2

3	9	7	4	1	6	5	2	8
1	8	5	9	2	7	4	6	3
4	2	6	3	8	5	9	7	1
5	1	2	7	9	3	8	4	6
7	6	9	8	5	4	3	1	2
8	3	4	2	6	1	7	9	5
2	5	3	1	7	9	6	8	4
9	4	8	6	3	2	1	5	7
6	7	1	5	4	8	2	3	9

PUZZLE #3

8	1	7	5	9	4	3	2	6
5	6	9	3	1	2	4	8	7
4	3	2	6	7	8	9	1	5
9	5	1	2	3	7	8	6	4
6	2	8	4	5	1	7	3	9
3	7	4	8	6	9	1	5	2
7	9	3	1	2	6	5	4	8
1	8	6	9	4	5	2	7	3
2	4	5	7	8	3	6	9	1

PUZZLE #4

7	4	6	1	5	2	3	9	8
1	3	5	9	8	7	6	2	4
9	8	2	3	4	6	1	7	5
4	7	3	6	9	1	8	5	2
6	5	9	8	2	3	4	1	7
8	2	1	5	7	4	9	6	3
5	6	4	2	3	9	7	8	1
3	9	8	7	1	5	2	4	6
2	1	7	4	6	8	5	3	9

PUZZLE #5

4	2	3	8	1	5	9	6	7
7	9	5	6	2	4	1	3	8
8	6	1	9	3	7	5	2	4
1	3	4	2	9	8	6	7	5
6	8	9	7	5	3	2	4	1
5	7	2	1	4	6	8	9	3
9	4	6	5	7	1	3	8	2
2	5	7	3	8	9	4	1	6
3	1	8	4	6	2	7	5	9

PUZZLE #6

2	1	3	4	7	8	5	9	6
6	5	7	2	3	9	8	4	1
4	9	8	1	5	6	7	2	3
8	4	1	7	6	2	3	5	9
7	2	9	5	4	3	6	1	8
5	3	6	8	9	1	2	7	4
9	8	5	6	2	4	1	3	7
3	6	2	9	1	7	4	8	5
1	7	4	3	8	5	9	6	2

PUZZLE #7

7	3	5	6	1	2	4	9	8
8	2	6	4	3	9	7	1	5
4	9	1	8	5	7	3	2	6
1	8	4	7	6	3	9	5	2
9	7	3	5	2	8	1	6	4
6	5	2	1	9	4	8	3	7
3	6	8	2	4	1	5	7	9
5	4	9	3	7	6	2	8	1
2	1	7	9	8	5	6	4	3

PUZZLE #8

7	9	8	4	6	3	1	5	2
2	1	3	9	5	7	4	6	8
4	6	5	2	8	1	7	3	9
8	7	1	5	3	2	9	4	6
9	3	4	6	1	8	5	2	7
5	2	6	7	9	4	8	1	3
6	5	2	8	4	9	3	7	1
3	8	7	1	2	5	6	9	4
1	4	9	3	7	6	2	8	5

PUZZLE #9

8	7	5	4	9	2	3	6	1
2	1	9	6	3	8	7	5	4
6	4	3	7	1	5	2	8	9
1	6	8	3	4	7	5	9	2
7	9	4	5	2	6	1	3	8
5	3	2	1	8	9	6	4	7
3	8	7	9	6	1	4	2	5
4	2	1	8	5	3	9	7	6
9	5	6	2	7	4	8	1	3

PUZZLE #10

6	9	5	7	1	8	4	2	3
8	2	7	4	3	6	1	9	5
4	1	3	2	5	9	6	8	7
1	6	4	8	7	5	9	3	2
5	3	8	9	2	1	7	4	6
9	7	2	6	4	3	5	1	8
2	5	1	3	6	4	8	7	9
3	4	9	5	8	7	2	6	1
7	8	6	1	9	2	3	5	4

PUZZLE #11

7	2	8	3	4	9	6	5	1
4	1	9	6	7	5	8	2	3
6	5	3	1	8	2	9	7	4
9	4	1	2	6	7	3	8	5
3	8	7	9	5	1	4	6	2
5	6	2	4	3	8	1	9	7
2	3	4	7	9	6	5	1	8
8	7	6	5	1	4	2	3	9
1	9	5	8	2	3	7	4	6

PUZZLE #12

1	4	7	6	2	5	8	9	3
8	9	3	1	4	7	5	2	6
6	2	5	3	9	8	7	4	1
3	8	4	5	7	6	2	1	9
7	1	2	8	3	9	4	6	5
5	6	9	4	1	2	3	8	7
4	7	6	2	5	1	9	3	8
9	3	1	7	8	4	6	5	2
2	5	8	9	6	3	1	7	4

PUZZLE #13

7	8	1	4	5	9	6	2	3
9	4	3	7	2	6	1	5	8
5	6	2	1	3	8	9	7	4
2	5	6	9	8	3	7	4	1
3	7	4	2	1	5	8	6	9
8	1	9	6	4	7	2	3	5
1	9	5	3	7	2	4	8	6
4	3	7	8	6	1	5	9	2
6	2	8	5	9	4	3	1	7

PUZZLE #14

7	8	1	4	5	9	6	2	3
9	4	3	7	2	6	1	5	8
5	6	2	1	3	8	9	7	4
2	5	6	9	8	3	7	4	1
3	7	4	2	1	5	8	6	9
8	1	9	6	4	7	2	3	5
1	9	5	3	7	2	4	8	6
4	3	7	8	6	1	5	9	2
6	2	8	5	9	4	3	1	7

PUZZLE #15

2	4	7	9	3	6	1	8	5
3	1	8	2	4	5	6	9	7
9	6	5	7	8	1	4	2	3
6	9	2	8	7	4	3	5	1
5	7	3	1	6	9	2	4	8
4	8	1	3	5	2	9	7	6
7	3	9	4	1	8	5	6	2
8	2	6	5	9	3	7	1	4
1	5	4	6	2	7	8	3	9

PUZZLE #16

9	1	4	3	8	6	5	7	2
3	7	5	2	9	4	8	1	6
6	8	2	1	5	7	4	9	3
7	2	8	6	1	3	9	5	4
5	6	3	8	4	9	1	2	7
1	4	9	5	7	2	3	6	8
4	3	1	7	2	5	6	8	9
2	5	6	9	3	8	7	4	1
8	9	7	4	6	1	2	3	5

PUZZLE #17

5	9	3	4	2	6	8	7	1
8	4	2	7	1	5	9	3	6
7	6	1	3	9	8	2	5	4
6	3	9	8	7	2	4	1	5
4	8	5	1	3	9	7	6	2
2	1	7	6	5	4	3	9	8
1	7	8	5	4	3	6	2	9
9	5	6	2	8	7	1	4	3
3	2	4	9	6	1	5	8	7

PUZZLE #18

7	8	6	4	3	1	5	9	2
2	9	3	7	8	5	6	4	1
1	4	5	2	6	9	7	8	3
3	1	7	6	2	4	8	5	9
4	2	9	5	7	8	3	1	6
6	5	8	9	1	3	4	2	7
9	3	1	8	4	7	2	6	5
8	7	2	1	5	6	9	3	4
5	6	4	3	9	2	1	7	8

PUZZLE #19

9	6	4	1	3	5	2	7	8
7	1	8	9	2	6	4	3	5
3	2	5	8	4	7	1	6	9
8	5	1	6	7	9	3	4	2
2	4	7	5	8	3	9	1	6
6	9	3	2	1	4	5	8	7
5	7	9	4	6	1	8	2	3
1	3	2	7	9	8	6	5	4
4	8	6	3	5	2	7	9	1

PUZZLE #20

7	8	5	1	2	9	6	4	3
3	9	1	7	6	4	2	8	5
6	4	2	3	5	8	9	1	7
4	2	7	9	1	3	8	5	6
5	3	8	6	4	7	1	9	2
9	1	6	5	8	2	7	3	4
2	7	3	8	9	5	4	6	1
8	6	4	2	3	1	5	7	9
1	5	9	4	7	6	3	2	8

WORD SEARCH
SOLUTIONS

PUZZLE #1

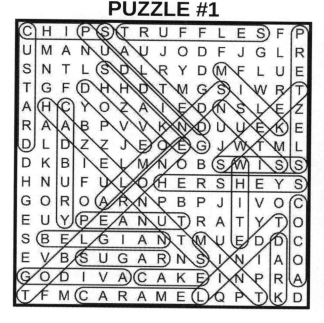

PUZZLE #2

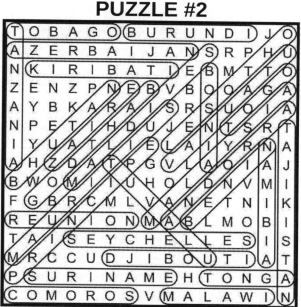

PUZZLE #3

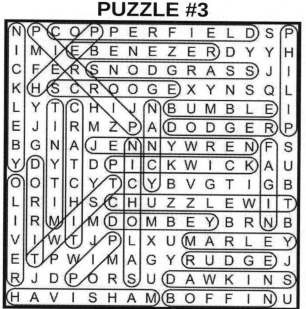

PUZZLE #4

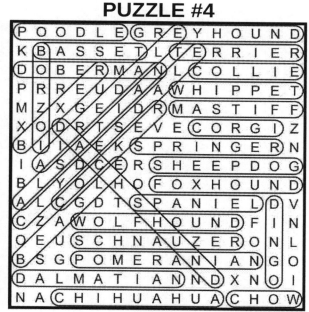

PUZZLE #5

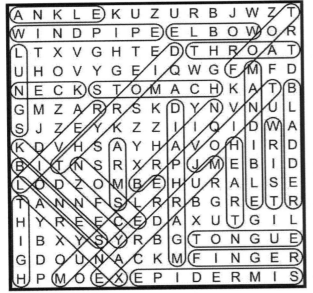

PUZZLE #6

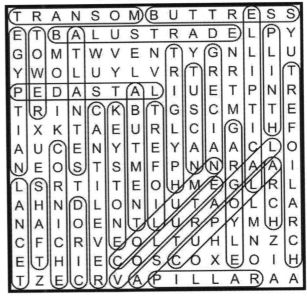

PUZZLE #7

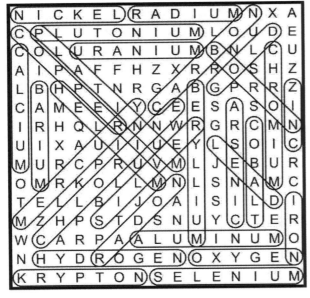

PUZZLE #8

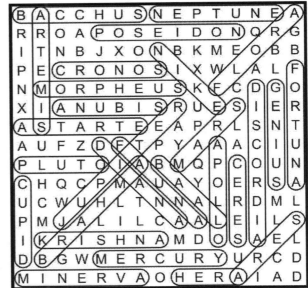

PUZZLE #9

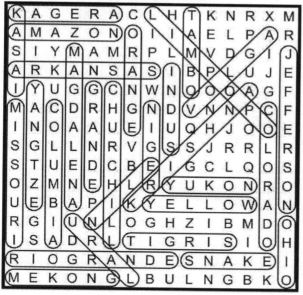

PUZZLE #10

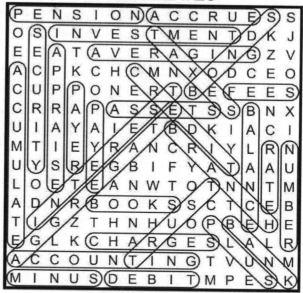

PUZZLE #11

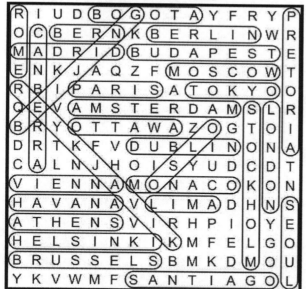

PUZZLE #12

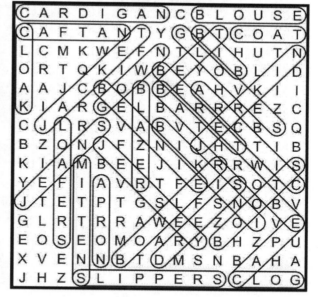

PUZZLE #13

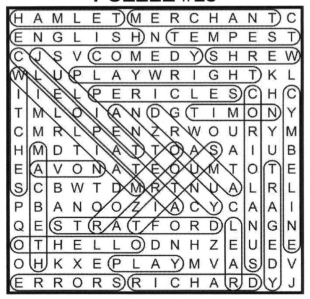

PUZZLE #14

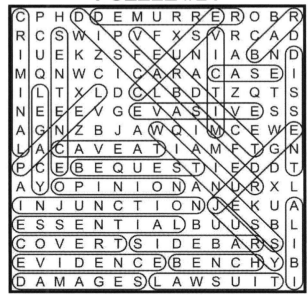

PUZZLE #15

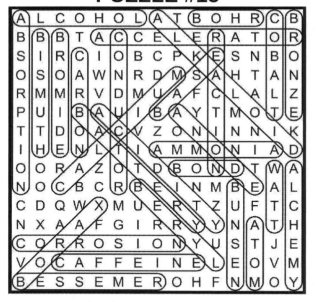

PUZZLE #16

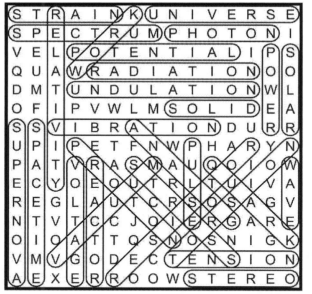

PUZZLE #17

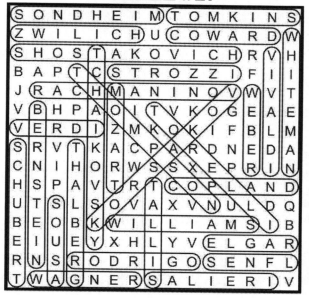

PUZZLE #18

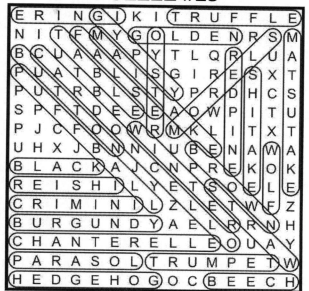

PUZZLE #19

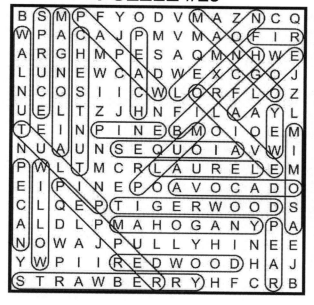

PUZZLE #20

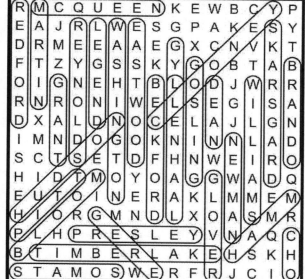

WORD JUMBLES
SOLUTIONS

PUZZLE 1

PARROT
THINK
PELLET
CHEST
CHIRP
MINTY

"Anyone who believes what a **cat tells him** deserves all he gets."
- Neil Gaiman

PUZZLE 2

BLATANT
KILTS
FLOCKS
FATTER
BAKED
YOUTH

"Dogs come when they're called; cats take a message and get **back to you later**." - Mary Bly

PUZZLE 3

BAKING
BURPS
MAILING
MOUSE
MINION
DATED

"Humans: No fur, no paws, no tail. They run away from mice. They never get enough sleep. How can you help but love such an **absurd animal**?" - Anonymous Cat

PUZZLE 4

BORAGE
WHIRL
MINCED
TANGY
SPRING
WITCH

"If a black cat crosses your path, it signifies that the animal is **going somewhere**." - Groucho Marx

PUZZLE 5

SOLVED
FLEET
FJORD
JOUST
MERRY
HOUR

"There is nothing noble in being superior to your fellow man; true nobility is being superior to **your former self**."

- Ernest Hemmingway

PUZZLE 6

FRIGHTS
BRIGHT
BERRY
HOUSES
PARTY
LOUSE

"Whether you believe you can do a thing or not, **you are right**. "
- Henry Ford

PUZZLE 7

ZEBRA
MUSCLE
ZESTY
WHOLE
PLUCKY
PLANTED

"Some men see things as they are and ask why. Others dream things that never were and **ask why not**."
- George Bernard Shaw

PUZZLE 8

QUESTS
MUSEUM
EATERY
SAUCIER
CLUED
CHURN

I like pigs. Dogs look up to us. Cats look down on us. Pigs **treat us as equals**. - Winston Churchill

PUZZLE 9

LACKEY
CRUMPET
POLISHES
YELLOW
MOOING
PLAID

"Never memorize something that **you can look up**."
- Albert Einstein

PUZZLE 10

RETRACT
DISTANCE
TRACK
SINCE
MARKET
HOSTILE

"Get your facts first, and then you _____ as much as you please. " - Mark Twain

PUZZLE 11

INKIER
YODELING
ROARING
HIRING
MEATY
YEARNS
BATTY

"Always forgive your enemies; **nothing annoys them** so much."
- Oscar Wilde

PUZZLE 12

PANSY
SOUPS
TAINTED
SPANISH
FRIDGE
GOING

"A lie gets halfway around the world before the truth has a chance to **get its pants on**." - Winston Churchill

PUZZLE 13

YAWN
MEANDER
WHIRR
NANNY
BOILED
MANAGE

"I like long walks, especially when they are taken by people **who annoy me**." - Fred Allen

PUZZLE 14

CADENCE
MELTED
AILING
PINTS
STAMINA

"I'm not crazy about reality, but it's still the only place to get **a decent meal**." - Groucho Marx

PUZZLE 15

WORTHY
DITHER
MORGUE
YARNS
WAITER
FOOT

"Never put off till tomorrow what may be done **day after tomorrow** just as well." - Mark Twain

PUZZLE 16

DELAYED
MOVER
ISLAND
MINGLE
LIDDED

"I **love deadlines**. I love the whooshing noise they make as they go by." - Douglas Adams

PUZZLE 17

YEARLY
ADMIRE
MYRIAD
MANY
DINER

"I never travel without **my diary**. One should always have something sensational to read in the train." - Oscar Wilde

PUZZLE 18

PILLER
TIGERS
GENDER
SNOOTS
IMPISH
GOURD

"I'm sure the universe is full of intelligent life. It's just been too **intelligent** to come here." - Arthur C. Clarke

PUZZLE 19

PRANKED
ROOTED
DEALT
HAPPY
HOMELY

"Outside of a dog, a book is man's best friend. Inside of a dog it's **too dark to read**." - Groucho Marx

PUZZLE 20

BELLY
WOOLLY
FLOOD
NOBBLE
FILLED
BRING

"A boy can learn a lot from a dog: obedience, loyalty, and the importance of turning around three times **before lying down**."
- Robert Benchley

WORD FIT
SOLUTIONS

PUZZLE #1

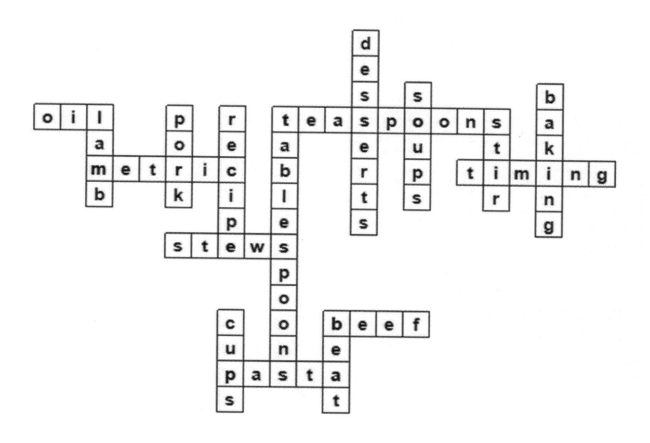

WORD FIT - PUZZLE #2

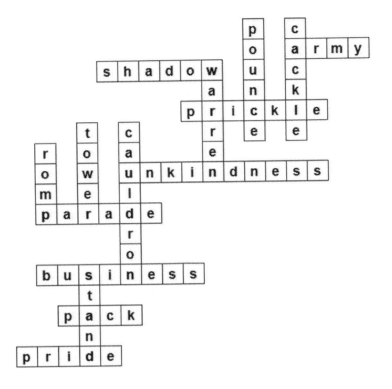

WORD FIT - PUZZLE #3

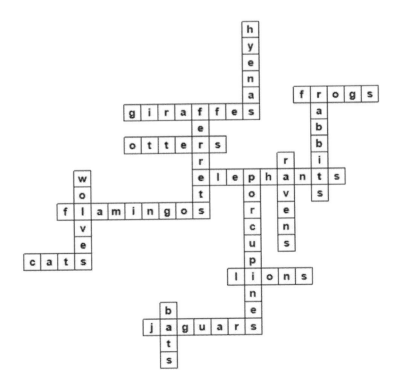

WORD FIT - PUZZLE #4

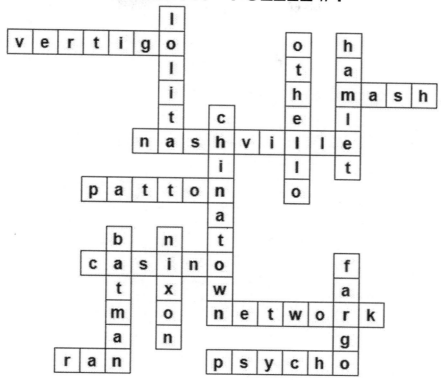

WORD FIT - PUZZLE #5

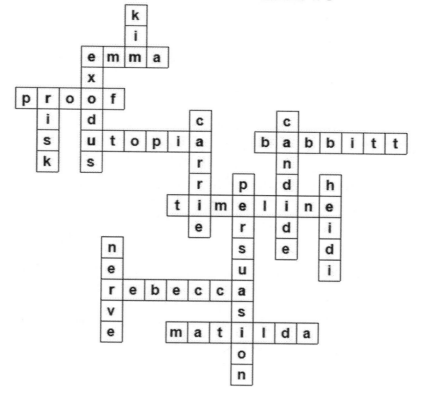

153

WORD FIT - PUZZLE #6

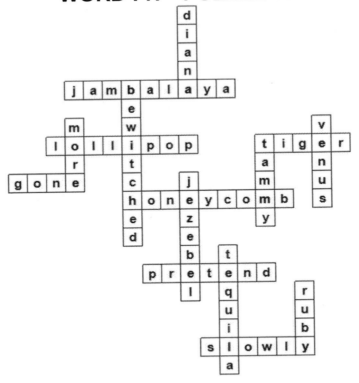

WORD FIT - PUZZLE #7

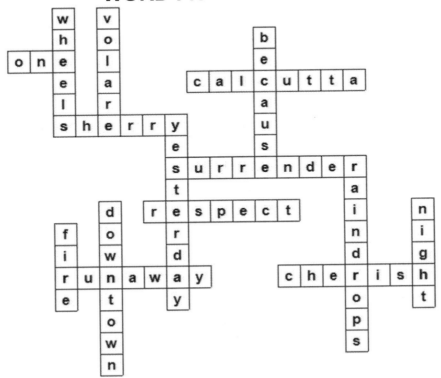

WORD FIT - PUZZLE #8

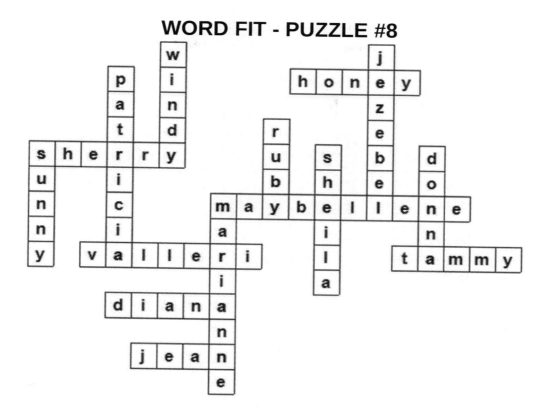

WORD FIT - PUZZLE #9

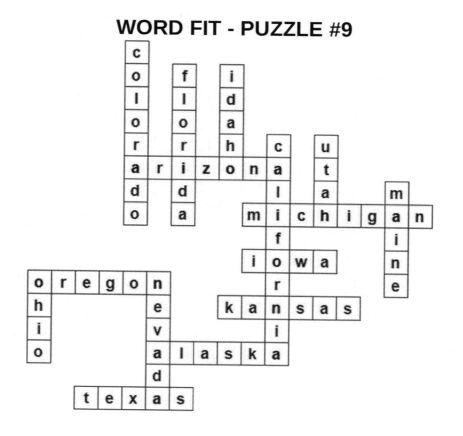

155

WORD FIT - PUZZLE #10

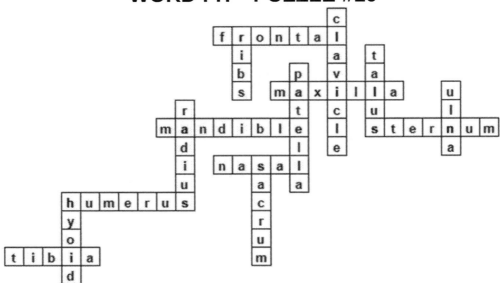

WORD FIT - PUZZLE #11

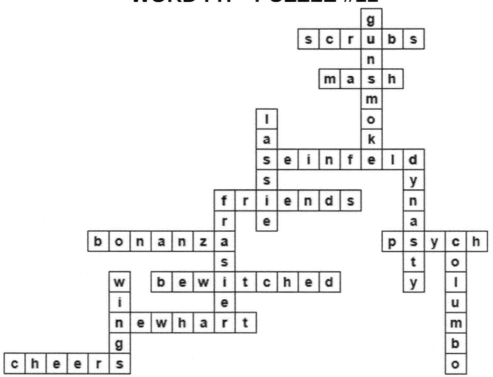

WORD FIT - PUZZLE #12

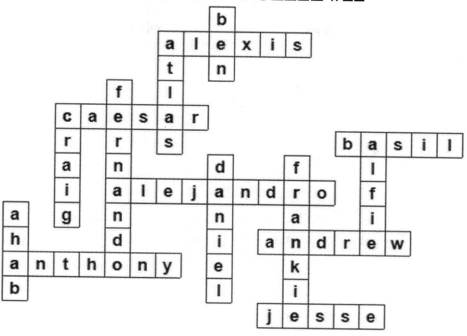

WORD FIT - PUZZLE #13

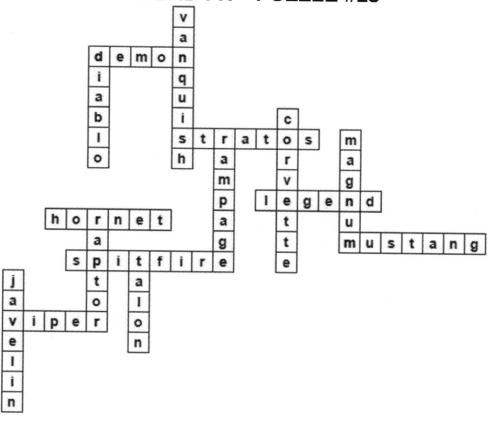

WORD FIT - PUZZLE #14

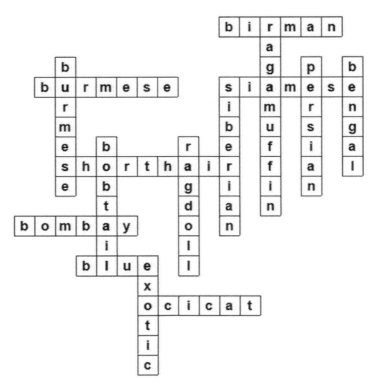

WORD FIT - PUZZLE #15

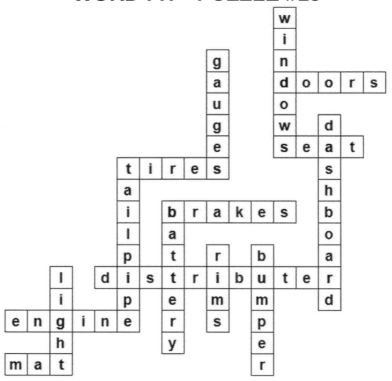

WORD FIT - PUZZLE #16

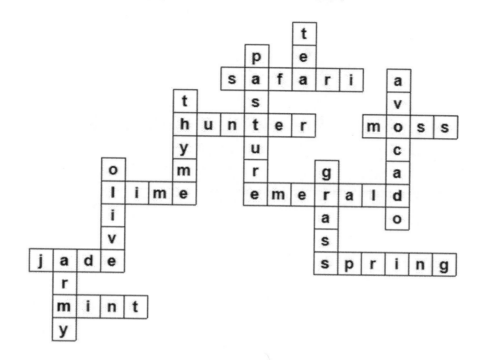

WORD FIT - PUZZLE #17

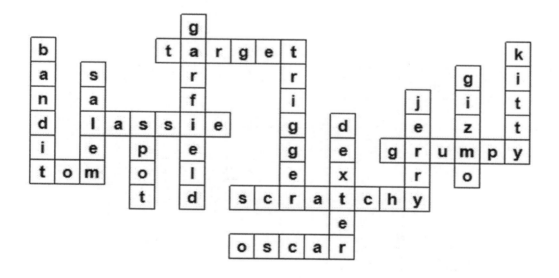

WORD FIT - PUZZLE #18

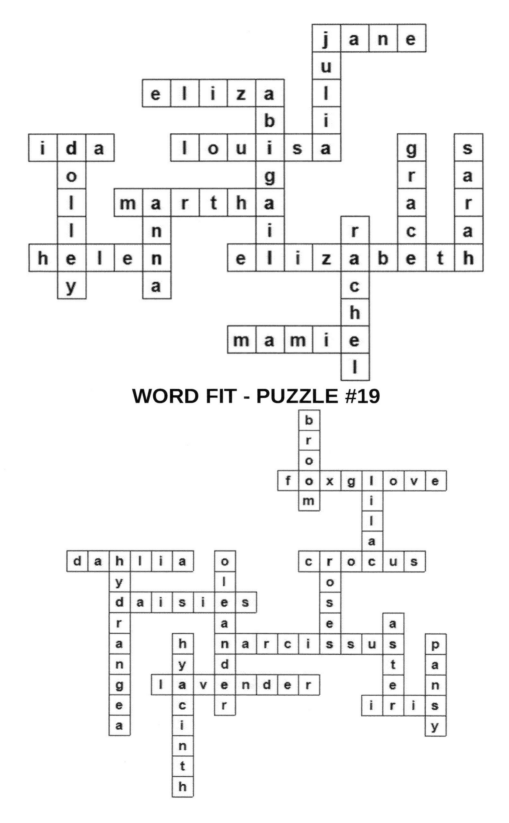

WORD FIT - PUZZLE #19

WORD FIT - PUZZLE #20

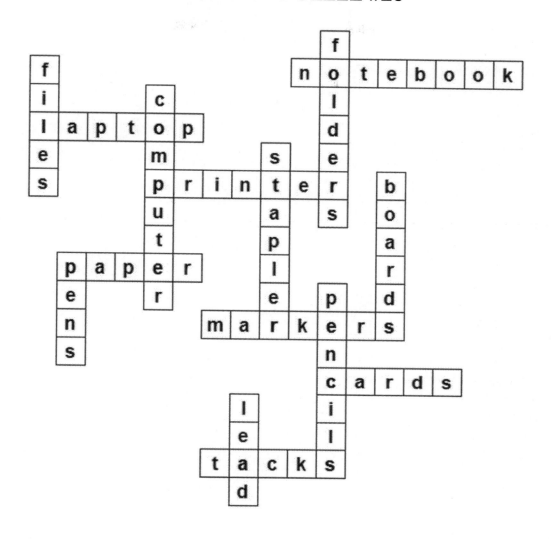

TOUGH TRIVIA
SOLUTIONS

1. St. Helena
2. Rasputin
3. A Whale Shark
4. Marcel Duchamp
5. Nepal
6. Polish
7. A
8. Nile or Amazon
9. Mount Everest
10. Coffee
11. Steel
12. Uranus
13. Republic of South Africa
14. An army
15. "O"
16. Dreamt
17. Jupiter
18. A murder
19. An unkindness
20. A blessing
21. America, not China as most people assume
22. Ursine
23. Cotton and linen
24. Cologne
25. Alarm clock
26. Prince Charles
27. Ear
28. Elephant
29. Sherlock Holmes
30. "42"
31. Da Vinci
32. 10, Downing Street
33. "1945"
34. In the beginning
35. Buddha
36. Big Ben
37. Genoa
38. "1865"
39. Miners
40. Michelangelo
41. Italy
42. Nairobi
43. Pacific
44. Addis Ababa
45. "64"
46. "4"
47. White
48. "10"
49. English
50. Paprika
51. Paul Newman and Robert Redford
52. Spain
53. Julius Caesar
54. Koran
55. "1954"
56. Frank Sinatra
57. Thomas Edison
58. Bonsai
59. Boxing
60. Red and Blue
61. Diamond
62. Thames

Dear Fellow Puzzle Lovers,

Thank you for purchasing this book. I hope it brings you hours of enjoyment.

As a small publishing company, reviews are the lifeblood of our continued success. If you could take a few minutes to leave us a review on Amazon it would be greatly appreciated.

www.oldtownpublishing.com/reviews

Thank you, Jenny

OTHER PUZZLE BOOKS RECOMMENDED FOR YOU

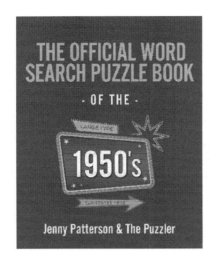

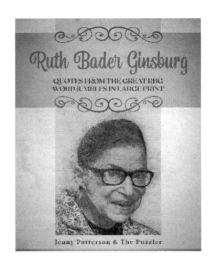

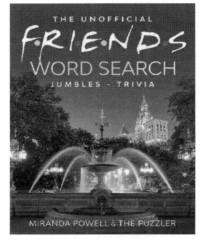

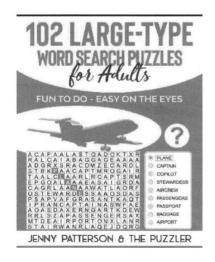

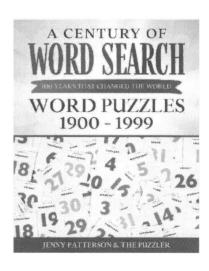

Available from Old Town Publishing

102 Large-Type Word Search Puzzles

A Kid's Christmas Word Search

A Year of Sudoku

A Century of Word Search

Adult Coloring Book - Animals

Brain Exercises for Seniors

Christmas Word Search Large-Print Puzzles

Crossword Puzzles for Kids Ages 6 - 8

Crosswords for Kids – Best Puzzle Book for Ages 8 and Up

Crosswords for Kids – Best Puzzle Book for Ages 9 and Up

Discover America – Word Search Puzzles for the 50 States

Easy-to-Read Crossword Puzzles for Adults

Everybody Loves Sudoku

Father's Day Puzzle Book

Giant Book of Crosswords for Kids

Giant Book of Word Puzzles for Kids

Happy Easter Word Puzzles

Happy Mother's Day Jumbles

Kid's Christmas Crosswords

Kid's Crossword Puzzle Book

Kid's Word Search Puzzle Book

Mad Words – Silly Fill-In Stories

Mad Words – My Weird Family

Mad Words – Summertime Fun

Mad Words – History of the World Part 1 1/2

Medium Crossword Puzzles for Adults – Large Print

My First 200 Sight Words

My Word Search Puzzle Book – Ages 7 and Up

Official Word Search Puzzle Book of the 1950s

Official Word Search Puzzle Book of the 1960s

Official Word Search Puzzle Book of the 1970s

Official Word Search Puzzle Book of the 1980s

Official Word Search Puzzle Book of the 1990s

Sudoku for Kids

The Best Kids Joke Book Ever

Wonderful Coloring and Writing Book

Word Jumbles for a Brighter Future

Word Jumbles Just for Women (Volume 1)

Word Jumbles Just for Women (Volume 2)

Word Puzzles for Cat Lovers

Word Puzzles for Dog Lovers

Word Puzzles for Early Readers

Word Puzzles for Mystery Lovers

Word Search Puzzles and More

Word Search Puzzles for Kids Ages 6 and Up

Word Search Puzzles for Kids Ages 8 and Up

Word Search Puzzles for Kids Ages 9 and Up

Word Search Puzzles Just for Women (Volume 1)

Word Search Puzzles Just for Women (Volume 2)

Manufactured by Amazon.ca
Bolton, ON